Preface

Incontinence is one of the commonest of nursing problems. Yet I could find no comprehensive nursing textbook on the subject when I started to work in an incontinence clinic. Information was available, but widely scattered throughout nursing, medical and paramedical books and journals. I have written *Nursing for Continence* to try to remedy this situation, in the hope that it might offer nurses a broad basis of knowledge about incontinence and their role in helping patients to achieve continence. The role of the nurse is central in the treatment and management of incontinent patients of all ages in both hospital and 'community' settings.

The book is written primarily for trained nurses working in clinical situations with patients who are, or who are at risk of becoming, incontinent. This includes 'general' nurses as well as those working in specialist areas such as care of the elderly, health visiting, mental handicap, district nursing and psychiatry. Such nurses have repeatedly asked me the same questions, wherever I have visited around the country – Why do older people become incontinent in hospital? Where can we start to promote continence when we have so many wet patients and so few staff? How can a patient with a persistently leaking catheter be helped? How do we persuade our Health Authority to purchase better quality incontinence aids? What is bladder training? The doctors are not interested in incontinence, what can we as nurses achieve alone?

I hope this book will answer these and many other questions. I hope that it will also be read by nurse teachers at the basic and post-basic level; by nurse learners wishing to pursue the topic in greater detail and by nurse administrators wishing to support their clinical colleagues in improving this aspect of care. Nurses taking the English National Board course 'Promotion of Continence and Management of Incontinence' will find it a useful starting-point for their in-depth studies. It should also be of interest to other professionals working with incontinent people – hospital doctors, general practitioners, physiotherapists, occupational therapists, social workers and those working with the elderly or disabled in social and welfare services and voluntary organisations.

I have not attempted to make the book exhaustively comprehensive – to do so would have made it unwieldy for most readers. I had to be selective, and chose to concentrate on describing nursing interventions in detail, leaving the reader to follow up the 'Reference and Further Reading' section of each chapter, as well as the general further reading in Appendix 3, for details of non-nursing interventions. The material presented is research-based where research has been done (which is by no means the case for all aspects covered). Reference is given to key pioneering research projects and to works that will lead the reader on to the available literature in the area.

I have presumed a systematic approach throughout, using the Nursing Process as a foundation for the delivery of nursing care. The book should give the nurse the sound basis of factual knowledge necessary to accurately assess her individual patient's problems and needs, to plan and implement the best available care to meet realistic goals, and to evaluate and adjust the care delivered as an ongoing process.

For simplicity I have referred to the nurse as 'she' and the patient as 'he' (except when discussing specifically female problems). Where examples of drug therapy are given, I have quoted an average adult dose, while recognising that some physicians use very different doses. All proprietary names are written with an initial capital letter, whilst non-proprietary (generic) names are written with small letters. Where incontinence aids are mentioned I have usually named specific products. This is not to claim that those mentioned are the only ones of their type available, or even necessarily that they are the best. The evaluative trials simply have not yet been done. My policy has been to select products which I have had experience of using and have found successful for the purposes mentioned. Appendix 1 lists the addresses of the manufacturers of the products named.

I owe thanks to many people for direct or indirect help with this book. Space will not permit me to name them all individually, but I would like to acknowledge an especial debt to: Stuart Stanton for his recognition of and support for the role of the specialist nurse, which first encouraged my interest in incontinence; to my friends and colleagues in the Association of Continence Advisors, who by so willingly sharing their expertise and experience have taught me much;

to David Lewin, who (albeit unwittingly) maintained my faith in nursing at an earlier stage; to Christine Hancock, who has been a supportive and imaginative CNO, and my other colleagues in Bloomsbury, particularly James Malone-Lee, Mandy Fader and Christine Budden at the Incontinence Clinic, St Pancras Hospital, London; to Helen White, Laila Orme, David Sines and Heather Butler-Gallie for advice on drafts of the manuscript; to Barbara Hyams for her illustrations and Pat Young for her copy-editing; to John Churchill for his enthusiasm and patience as a publisher and for recognising the importance of continence; to Enid Mills, my mother, for the time and care she took in her faultless typing of the manuscript; to Kingsley Norton, my husband, for believing that I could do it and allowing me the space in which to try, as well as his careful scrutiny of the result and the addition of the commas. Finally I would like to thank the many patients, and their families and carers, who have made this such a worthwhile and rewarding speciality to work in.

C.N.

Contents

PREFACE   iii

1   THE PROBLEM OF INCONTINENCE   1
    What is Incontinence?   2
    Who is Incontinent?   4
    Attitudes and Incontinence   6

2   THE DEVELOPMENT OF CONTINENCE, AND CAUSES
    OF INCONTINENCE   9
    The Baby's Bladder   9
      Acquisition of continence   10
    The 'Normal' Adult Bladder   12
    Causes of Urinary Incontinence   13

3   ASSESSMENT AND INVESTIGATION OF URINARY
    INCONTINENCE   27
    Presentation   27
    History   28
    Urodynamic studies   45

4   TREATING AND MANAGING INCONTINENCE   67
    Nursing Management and Advice   67
    The Role of the Doctor   75
      Drug therapy   75
      Surgery   78
    The Contribution of Other Team Members   79
    Bladder Training   80

5   INCONTINENCE IN CHILDHOOD   93
    Toilet Training   94
    Persistent Diurnal Incontinence   96
    Nocturnal Enuresis (Bedwetting)   98
    Congenital Abnormalities   106

Nursing For Continence

Christine Norton
MA, SRN

BEACONSFIELD PUBLISHERS LTD
Beaconsfield, Bucks, England

First published in 1986
Reprinted in 1989

British Library Cataloguing in Publication Data

Norton, Christine
Nursing for continence.
1. Urine — Incontinence — Nursing
2. Feces — Incontinence — Nursing
I. Title
610.73'69   RC921.I5

ISBN 0–906584–15–9

Medical illustrations by Barbara Hyams.
Phototypeset by Prima Graphics, Camberley, Surrey in 10 on 12 point Times.
Printed in Great Britain at the University Press, Oxford.

6   **FEMALE INCONTINENCE**   109
    Genuine Stress Incontinence   109
    Urinary Fistula   121
    Incontinence and Sexual Activity   122
    Incontinence in Pregnancy   122
    Occlusive Devices   123

7   **MALE INCONTINENCE**   128
    Prostatic Hypertrophy   128
    Carcinoma of the Prostate   132
    Urethral Stricture   132
    Bladder-Neck Obstruction   133
    Post-Micturition Dribbling   133
    Post-Prostatectomy Incontinence   135
    Control of Incontinence: the Penile Clamp   139

8   **INCONTINENCE AND THE ELDERLY**   141
    'Victorian Decency'   142
    The Physiological Effects of Ageing on Continence   144
    Attitudes and the Importance of the Environment   150
    Emotional and Psychological Factors   151
    Treatment of Incontinence in the Elderly   152
    Incontinence in Terminal Illness   153
    The Elderly Mentally Infirm   154

9   **AIDS TO CONTINENCE FOR THE PHYSICALLY DISABLED**   162
    Continence in Public Places   162
    Lavatory Design for the Disabled   163
    Alternatives to the Lavatory   166
    Clothing   171

10 **THE NEUROGENIC BLADDER**   174
    Sites of Neurological Damage   174
    Investigations   177
    Management   177
    Management of the Bladder After Spinal Injury   190

11 **FACTORS RELATED TO LOCATION**   192
    Home Care   192
    Residential and Hospital Care   201

12 **TOILET-TRAINING THE MENTALLY HANDICAPPED**   208
    Training Methods   210
    Baseline Observation   213
    The Training Programme   215
    Containment   217

13 **THE USE OF INCONTINENCE AIDS**   219
    Selection of Incontinence Aids   219
    Assessment   224
    Pads and Pants   226
    Male Appliances   236
    Bed Protection   243

14 **FAECAL INCONTINENCE**   247
    Faecal Continence   247
    The Causes of Faecal Incontinence   250
    Prevention of Faecal Incontinence   262
    Intractable Faecal Incontinence   263
    Faecal Incontinence in Children   263
    Faecal Incontinence in Dementia   265

15 **CATHETERISATION**   267
    Indwelling Urethral (Foley) Catheters   267
        Management of the short-term indwelling catheter   281
        Long-term indwelling catheter management   283
    Suprapubic Catheters   292

16 **THE NURSE AND THE CONTINENCE ADVISER**   295
    Continence – Every Nurse's Business   295
    The Development of Continence Advisers   297
    The Scope of a Continence Adviser   299

    APPENDIX 1   Addresses of Manufacturers and Suppliers   306

    APPENDIX 2   Useful Addresses   307

    APPENDIX 3   General Further Reading   307

Chapter 1

The Problem of Incontinence

Incontinence is one of the most unpleasant and distressing symptoms an individual can suffer. Those affected often feel embarrassed, ashamed, and alone. Most incontinent people hide their problem from society, from their family and friends, even from themselves. From the playground to the geriatric ward, incontinence attracts ridicule and blame, the sufferer is often ostracised and avoided. Health care professionals, whether nurses, doctors or paramedical workers, usually see only the tip of a vast iceberg of misery and distress.

Many professionals are profoundly ignorant about the causes and management of incontinence and are guilty of passive acceptance of the symptom in those who come under their care. It has largely been ignored as a research topic until very recently, and as yet there are very few clinics or resources to help the incontinent. With nowhere to turn for assistance, the majority of incontinent people attempt to cope alone or with the help of long-suffering relatives.

There are signs of change in this gloomy situation. Both the public and professionals are talking more about the subject. It is now being discussed in the media, a few articles in women's magazines and in occasional television and radio programmes. Chemists advertise incontinence aids rather than hide them under the counter. Study days, seminars and courses are becoming widespread and are often over-subscribed. Incontinence is coming to be seen as a 'respectable' symptom, and in spite of a feeling of shame, more people are seeking help. It is evident that in many instances incontinence will respond to appropriate treatment and can often be cured completely. Where cure is not attained, good management can enable the incontinent person to live a 'normal' life. To be incontinent no longer means inevitable discomfort and embarrassment.

At one time incontinence was seen largely as a 'nursing' problem, the only appropriate interventions being for the nurse to keep the patient as clean and comfortable as possible and to prevent pressure

1

sores developing. These aspects are important, but do not comprise comprehensive management. A nurse can now approach incontinence much more positively than in the days when the only equipment available was a mop and an underpad, and 'regular toileting' the only regime thought suitable. The wide range of nursing interventions and equipment available are not as yet well known or used; although there is still a long way to go, nurses are now in a position to see incontinence as a nursing challenge rather than as a problem to be tolerated.

Incontinence cannot be left to nurses alone. Many other professions are realising this and developing their own special skills for helping. This book aims to highlight the role of the nurse within the context of a multidisciplinary team approach to incontinence.

WHAT IS INCONTINENCE?

Is this a ridiculous question to ask a nurse? Every nurse has had to deal with incontinence at some time in her career, and recognises only too well the wet bed, the puddle on the floor, and the tell-tale odour. Some nurses deal with incontinence many times each day. Yet how many could offer a clear definition of the term? 'Continence' is not an absolute concept. We all have to pass urine and faeces. Incontinence is not to do with the fact of excretion, but with its location and timing. Continence very much depends on society's rules for acceptable excretion. Those who cannot or will not abide by these rules are thereby defined as 'incontinent'.

At the simplest level, continence is passing urine and faeces only in the socially accepted place, and incontinence is excretion in the 'wrong' place. The rules are often quite arbitrary. The person who parks his car in a lay-by at night and relieves himself behind a tree is not normally classed as incontinent, because this is an accepted practice. To do the same in broad daylight in a crowded street invites at best public censure, at worst arrest and criminal proceedings. If urine or faeces are passed in the wrong place, whether into clothing, in bed or onto the ground, or into the wrong receptacle, this will usually be called 'incontinence'.

Some definitions note the fact that incontinence is 'involuntary' – the individual cannot help it. The distinction between voluntary and involuntary excretion in the wrong place is largely academic and the results are similar. The International Continence Society takes the definition a step further and defines urinary incontinence as 'a

2

condition where involuntary loss of urine is a social or hygienic problem . . .' This emphasises that the results of the event should be considered. Incontinence is the state where passing urine in the 'wrong' place has become a problem (whether to the individual or those around him). This may vary between people and circumstances. What amounts to a problem for one person may be ignored by another. No absolute values can be given for the volume or frequency of loss that will constitute 'incontinence' for any individual (although a consistent definition is necessary for research purposes and should always be stated explicitly for a research study).

The general public's interpretation of the term 'incontinence' is often different from the medically accepted usage. Many people would only use the term to describe total lack of control. Often it is used pejoratively to reflect on the character or self-control of the incontinent person – misunderstandings between professional and patient can easily arise because of this. The individual who denies he is incontinent may admit to 'wetting' or 'leaking'.

Incontinence can have widespread ramifications for the individual, for those around him, and for society. It creates many physical and psychosocial problems for all sufferers. Some, possibly most, cope reasonably well with little apparent disruption of lifestyle. For those who cope less well it can become the dominant factor in their life. For a few it can tip the balance between living independently and needing residential care. Those close to incontinent people, whether relatives, friends, or professional carers, are usually also affected. On occasion the relationship may be reduced to an endless round of washing and changing, which becomes an intolerable burden.

The costs of incontinence to the country as a whole are vast. The health and social services spend huge amounts on the problem. Incontinence aids alone were estimated in 1982 to cost £36 million (Royal College of Nursing), and this takes no account of services (such as home help, laundry, residential care), prolonged hospital stay and – possibly the most neglected item – nursing time and morale. In both hospital and community far too many nurses spend far too much of their time and energy dealing with the results. It is surely time to re-think the nursing approach to incontinence and come up with some more positive and therapeutic answers.

WHO IS INCONTINENT?

It is commonly supposed that incontinence is a problem exclusive to the elderly. The common image is of a confused, dependent, elderly woman, usually in a long-stay geriatric hospital. The physically or mentally disabled, and possibly the enuretic boy, may also come to mind. Very few people, whether lay or professional, realise that incontinence can affect almost anyone. Far from being a problem confined to the elderly or disabled, it is common in people of all ages, both fit and disabled. The prevalence does increase with age and disability, but the majority of incontinent people are neither elderly nor disabled. Most live at home and lead otherwise 'normal' lives, with incontinence being their major health problem.

Until recently, evidence about who suffers from incontinence was patchy and inconclusive. Table 1.1 shows the results obtained from a large-scale prevalence study based on over 18,000 replies to a postal questionnaire conducted in several locations in the UK (Thomas et al., 1980). The definition of 'regular' incontinence was 'involuntary excretion or leakage of urine in inappropriate places or at inappropriate times twice or more a month, regardless of the quantity of urine lost'. The table shows that in those under 65 years old, urinary incontinence was far commoner in women, and that this difference tended to equalise in the older age-groups. Nearly twice as many people reported 'occasional' urinary incontinence occurring less than twice per month. Overall, 72.4% of women and 89.2% of men said they were *never* incontinent – i.e. one in four women and one in ten men had some incontinence, and for around 5% of the total population this was regular.

In the same study, a figure was obtained for 'recognised' incontinence by asking the health, social, and voluntary services in the same areas to identify people they knew to be incontinent. Table 1.2 shows the results. By comparing this with Table 1.1 it is obvious that only a tiny proportion of those with incontinence were presenting for help with it. Of those people with recognised incontinence, one-half of the total

Table 1.1:   Prevalence of Regular Urinary Incontinence

Sex	Age 15–64 years	Age 65 years +
Male	1.6%	6.9%
Female	8.5%	11.6%

('Regular' = twice or more per month)   (Thomas et al., 1980)

Table 1.2:   Prevalence of 'Recognised' Urinary Incontinence

Sex	Age 15–64 years	Age 65 years +
Male	0.1%	1.3%
Female	0.2%	2.5%

('Recognised' = known to be incontinent by health, social, or voluntary services)

(Thomas et al., 1980)

were resident in long-stay institutions, so the vast majority of incontinent people outside long-stay care are unknown to the health and social services. It seems that about only one in ten incontinent people seek any help.

Of the total number of people in the questionnaire reporting incontinence, one in five were judged to have a moderate or severe problem, involving extra laundry or expenses, use of pads, some restriction of activities, and possibly requiring help from others. Of those with a moderate or severe problem, less than one-half were receiving any services.

Extrapolations from these results suggest that between two and three million people in the UK may be incontinent of urine at least twice a month. Care should be taken not to presume that all these people see their incontinence as a problem. Four-fifths of this total had only minimal or slight incontinence, which may or may not be seen as a problem depending on the characteristics of each individual. About 1% of adults are thought to have regular nocturnal enuresis.

Faecal incontinence is less common than urinary incontinence and affects about 0.5% of adults – yet even this involves a very large number of individuals.

The prevalence of incontinence among people in institutional care should be easier to discover, yet reports vary so widely that it is difficult to generalise. Studies have used very different (and often unquoted) definitions of incontinence. In hospitals, probably 80% of all incontinent people are in acute or general wards, with only 20% of the overall total being in long-stay or continuing care wards (Egan et al., 1983). However, in long-stay wards the *proportion* of patients who are incontinent is much higher than on acute wards. Between 13% and 48% of patients in beds labelled 'geriatric' (acute, rehabilitation, and long-stay combined) are incontinent (Milne, 1976). Between 30% and 40% of people in long-stay geriatric care and 30% to 50% in long-stay psychogeriatric care are frequently incontinent (Gilleard, 1981).

Some studies have suggested that only 10% of psychogeriatric long-stay patients are totally continent (McLaren, 1981). In residential homes 17% of residents are reported to be incontinent of urine (Masterton et al., 1980).

It must be noted that these overall percentages disguise huge variations locally. Although useful for planning services they do little to predict how many incontinent people there are in an individual home or hospital. In some there is very litle incontinence; in others virtually everyone is incontinent. The reasons for these variations are many and complex.

Is all this incontinence unavoidable or inevitable? Probably not. Many types of incontinence are curable; research suggests that complete continence is attainable, for example, for 90% of women with stress incontinence, and 80% with urge incontinence, if accurate diagnosis is made prior to treatment. It is likely that many more people could benefit than are at present receiving treatment. The potential of preventive measures is still largely unexplored.

ATTITUDES AND INCONTINENCE

Attitudes towards incontinence present a major problem in tackling it. As nurses we can usefully begin by examining our own attitudes.

Passive acceptance of incontinence, as an inevitable part of working in certain situations or with certain patient groups, is common. With increased knowledge and awareness this is gradually changing towards a more positive problem-solving approach to each individual. With the move towards individualised patient-centred delivery of nursing care, incontinence can be identified as a symptom of a patient with a unique combination of problems, needs and potentials, rather than an inevitable part of working with the elderly.

Incontinence often arouses as much revulsion in a nurse as in anyone else. Few people enjoy dealing with other people's excreta, or even with their own. Yet nurses are expected, right from the beginning of their training, to ignore their own automatic reactions. This must be one of the most unpleasant aspects of nursing, and is usually what members of the public mean when they say that they could never be a nurse, or that nurses are wonderful for putting up with the things they have to do for people. Nurses are not encouraged to discuss or express their emotions about this aspect of their work. A nurse must expect and accept incontinence as part of the job, and get on and deal with it. Feelings of distaste are considered unworthy and best ignored – 'you will soon get used to it'. It is this very 'getting used to it' that leads to a tendency to deal with incontinence as quickly as possible, usually in a manner which detaches the individual nurse from the personal reality of the situation. Incontinence is cleared away and forgotten so that the nurse may move on to a pleasanter aspect of care – until the next time. This, combined with the patient's embarrassment, can lead to a situation of 'mutual pretence' (Schwartz, 1977) between nurse and patient that nothing abnormal has occurred. Neither nurse nor patient talks about the incontinence, even while it is actually being cleared up. The nurse wishes to spare the patient's feelings, and the patient is ashamed and assumes it cannot be helped. It is seldom openly and frankly discussed. Alternatively, the nurse may take a patronising attitude, reassuring the patient that it does not matter and that it happens all the time – 'Don't worry, dear, we have plenty more sheets in the cupboard'. Neither the pretence nor the bland platitudes help to get to the cause of the incontinence.

Nurses need to be able to discuss their own feelings more openly, without fear of censure. The nurse may feel embarrassed, both for herself and her patient. She may feel guilty, since incontinence is sometimes interpreted as a sign of 'bad' nursing care. Anger with a patient is particularly difficult to admit. Anger may result from the extra, unpleasant work created by incontinence, or because the patient is felt to be lazy, or wetting on purpose to gain attention or to annoy the staff. Many of these feelings – revulsion, guilt, embarrassment, and anger – are understandable. They should be admitted and examined openly, rather than repressed as unworthy of a professional nurse, if the nurse is to be able to view the patient's incontinence objectively and plan a rational care regime. Constructive assessment can only result from the nurse being aware of her own attitudes to the problem.

Nurses have a tradition of coping, whatever the situation, of putting up with problems however great or unpleasant, and making the best they can of them. Incontinence has always been coped with, after a fashion. For the sake of our incontinent patients, as well as for nurses themselves, it is time to look at how the situation could be altered. Nursing as a profession has a responsibility to patients and their families to use the best available expertise in providing care, both for the promotion of continence and the management of incontinence, and in fostering a positive approach amongst carers.

REFERENCES AND FURTHER READING

Egan, M., Plymat, K., Thomas, T., Meade, T., 1983. 'Incontinence in patients in two district general hospitals'. *Nursing Times*, 79, 5, 22–24.

Gilleard, C. J., 1981. 'Incontinence in the hospitalised elderly'. *Health Bulletin*, 39, 1, 58–61.

McLaren, S. M., McPherson, F. M., Sinclair, F., Ballinger, B. R., 1981. 'Prevalence and severity of incontinence among hospitalised female psycho-geriatric patients'. *Health Bulletin*, 39, 3, 157–161.

Masterton, G., Holloway, E. M., Timbury, G. C., 1980. 'The prevalence of incontinence in local authority homes for the elderly'. *Health Bulletin*, 38, 2, 62–64.

Milne, J. S., 1976. 'Prevalence of incontinence in the elderly age groups'. In: Willington, F., (ed.). *Incontinence in the Elderly*. Academic Press, London.

Royal College of Nursing, 1982. *The Problem of Promoting Continence*, RCN, London.

Schwartz, D. R., 1977. 'Personal point of view – a report of 17 elderly patients with a persistent problem of urinary incontinence'. *Health Bulletin*, 35, 4, 197–204.

Thomas, T. M., Plymat, K. R., Blannin, J., Meade, T. W., 1980. 'Prevalence of urinary incontinence'. *British Medical Journal*, 281, 1243–1245.

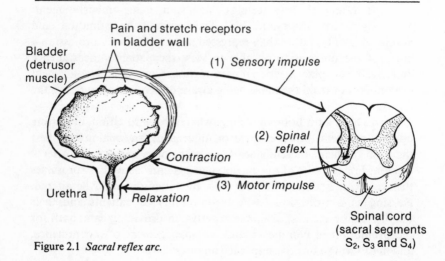

Figure 2.1 *Sacral reflex arc.*

Chapter 2

The Development of Continence, and Causes of Incontinence

None of us is born continent. Continence is a skill acquired, at a variable age, and retained often only with difficulty. This chapter aims to provide a framework for understanding, in a simplified form, the mechanism of continence and the most common causes of incontinence. Subsequent chapters explain in greater depth many of the types of incontinence introduced here.

Any nurse who wishes to help incontinent patients needs a thorough grasp of the normal functioning of the bladder and the ways in which it may become disordered. This will make it possible to assess the causes of an individual's incontinence (see Chapter 3) and set appropriate and realistic goals during care planning.

THE BABY'S BLADDER

The bladder of the newborn baby is controlled by a sacral reflex arc (Figure 2.1, opposite). As the bladder fills with urine (which drains from the kidneys via the ureters), stretch and pain receptors in the bladder wall send sensory impulses to the sacral bladder centre in the spinal cord (located in sacral segments S_2, S_3, and S_4). When these impulses become strong and persistent enough a spinal reflex arc is completed, and motor impulses cause a bladder contraction, co-ordinated with relaxation of the urethral sphincter. The bladder empties completely. The whole filling and emptying cycle is then repeated. Babies are therefore not continuously wet, but 'incontinent' in episodes throughout the 24-hour period. At this stage the immature central nervous system is incapable of either consciously appreciating or voluntarily controlling this cycle.

ACQUISITION OF CONTINENCE

Continence is acquired by the interaction of two processes – socialisation of the infant, and maturation of the central nervous system. Potty-training is dealt with in Chapter 5. Suffice it to say here that without society's expectation of continence, and without broadly accepted definitions of correct behaviour, the whole concept of 'incontinence' would be meaningless.

As the central nervous system matures with age, the baby is increasingly aware of its various bodily functions, including bladder emptying. With practice, voluntary control becomes possible, just as control of limb movements becomes more purposeful. Figure 2.2 shows that the sensory messages from the bladder are relayed, via several intermediate centres, to the cerebral cortex, where the micturition control centre is situated in the frontal lobe. As maturation progresses the infant is able to interpret these signals as indicating a full bladder; and, with practice, to initiate inhibitory motor impulses

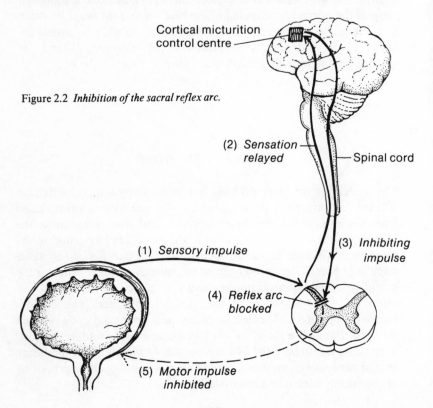

Figure 2.2 *Inhibition of the sacral reflex arc.*

Cortical micturition control centre

(2) *Sensation relayed*

Spinal cord

(1) *Sensory impulse*

(3) *Inhibiting impulse*

(4) *Reflex arc blocked*

(5) *Motor impulse inhibited*

to block the completion of the sacral reflex arc, and thus prevent micturition. Continence involves an active inhibition of nerve impulses, not merely the passive absence of micturition. Eventually the child learns to delay micturition reliably until the appropriate time and place are reached. The cerebral inhibition is then removed, the sacral reflex arc is completed, and the bladder contracts and empties (Figure 2.3). Micturition is co-ordinated by several very complex feedback loops between the bladder and brain stem. These ensure that bladder contraction is simultaneous with sphincter relaxation, and that voiding continues until the bladder is completely empty.

With time, this control no longer involves continuous conscious effort between the first sensation of bladder filling and micturition. Continence becomes subconscious and automatic under most circumstances.

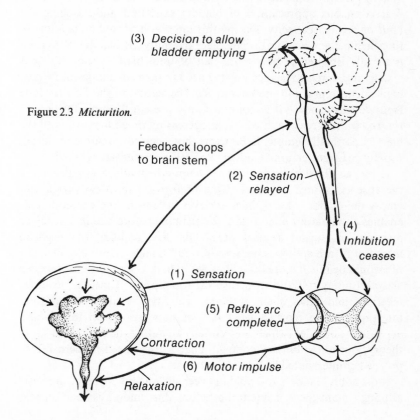

Figure 2.3 *Micturition.*

(3) *Decision to allow bladder emptying*

Feedback loops to brain stem

(2) *Sensation relayed*

(4) *Inhibition ceases*

(1) *Sensation*

(5) *Reflex arc completed*

Contraction

(6) *Motor impulse*

Relaxation

THE 'NORMAL' ADULT BLADDER

Bladder control and function is taken for granted by most people from an early age, and few adults pay it any attention. Indeed, few people are able to give an accurate account of how often they pass urine, until something goes wrong with control.

The boundaries of 'normality' are quite wide, and possibly 'normal' should be defined as the absence of any problem for each individual. Most people empty the bladder between three and six times in twenty-four hours. Some people do so more or less often than this and would still class themselves as normal. Most people seldom have to get up at night, but a few always have to get up once. Urgency (having to rush to the lavatory) should be rare, and only experienced if bladder sensations have been ignored for too long or if fluid intake has been excessive. Generally the bladder has a very effective early warning system – most people have a margin of one to two hours between the first conscious appreciation of bladder sensation and reaching the limit of bladder capacity. During this interval it should be possible to find the time and an appropriate place to empty the bladder. Sensation is usually first felt at about one-half of total bladder capacity. It is usually registered consciously as the need to take advantage of the next convenient opportunity to pass urine. The sensation should then fade from consciousness – it is not constantly present until micturition. It returns with increasing intensity, at decreasing time intervals, until the bladder is finally emptied. Between these periodic reminders it can usually be forgotten until bladder capacity is very nearly reached.

A very useful skill is the ability to empty the bladder at will, even in the absence of any sensation of the need to do so. Most people can empty the bladder at any time, however little urine there is in it. This enables anticipatory micturition, for example before a long journey or meeting, or during a meal break, thereby avoiding the need to interrupt future activities because of a full bladder. Ordinary civilised life would be much more difficult if we all had to wait until the bladder was absolutely full and then rush off to empty it. Cinemas, lectures, meetings and other such structured activities would be constantly interrupted. The remarkable ability of most people to inhibit and activate the bladder (which is essentially an automatic organ and so, in theory, outside voluntary control), enables organised modern life to proceed uninterrupted by 'calls of nature'.

Most adult bladders will hold between 400ml and 600ml at capacity, although many people micturate before this volume is reached. No incontinence should occur at any time, even if micturition has been delayed and urgency is severe, including during strenuous exercise and while asleep.

CAUSES OF URINARY INCONTINENCE

There are many reasons why some people never acquire the control described above, or why it may break down at some point in life, and any classification of the causes is necessarily arbitrary. However, some scheme for considering the causes is needed, and in this book they are divided into three broad categories: physiological bladder dysfunction; factors directly influencing bladder functioning; and factors affecting the individual's ability to cope with bladder function. Table 2.1 summarises the major types of incontinence and the most common associated symptoms. It should be remembered that these categories are intimately interrelated and that they often overlap.

Table 2.1: Common Causes Of Urinary Incontinence

Physiological Bladder Dysfunction	*Usual Symptoms*
Detrusor instability	Frequency, urgency, urge incontinence
Genuine stress incontinence	Incontinence upon physical exertion
Outflow obstruction	Dribbling overflow incontinence, nocturia
Atonic bladder	Dribbling overflow incontinence, recurrent UTI
Factors Influencing Bladder Function	*Usual Symptoms*
Urinary tract infection	Frequency, dysuria, urgency and urge incontinence
Faecal impaction	Voiding difficulty with overflow incontinence or stress incontinence
Drug therapy	Various
Endocrine disorder	Various
Miscellaneous bladder pathology	Various
Factors Affecting Ability to Cope with Bladder	*Usual Symptoms*
Immobility	Urge incontinence or 'voluntary' wetting
Environment	Various
Mental function	Behavioural incontinence
Emotions	Urge incontinence or apathetic incontinence
Carers	'Institutional' incontinence

Nursing for Continence

PHYSIOLOGICAL BLADDER DYSFUNCTION

The causes of incontinence which fall into this category involve an abnormality in actual bladder function. The bladder, at its most basic, only has two functions: to hold urine until the correct time for micturition, and then to expel it completely. The first two causes described here involve a failure to hold urine reliably during bladder filling; the second two involve a failure to expel it completely and leave no residue after micturition.

Most, but not all, people who are incontinent have some underlying degree of bladder dysfunction. For some it is the only cause of their incontinence. For others it is a necessary, but not sufficient, predisposing reason. Alone, it does not explain entirely why they are wet – and many are actually precipitated into frank incontinence by the coincidence of another problem from one of the other categories described below. A few incontinent people do not have any abnormality of bladder functioning and are wet solely for reasons discussed on pages 18–25.

Four basic types of bladder dysfunction may be distinguished. These are: detrusor instability; genuine stress incontinence; outflow obstruction; and an atonic bladder.

Detrusor instability

Detrusor instability (which may also be referred to as bladder instability, or the unstable bladder) is a condition characterised by involuntary bladder (detrusor muscle) contractions during bladder filling. The normal inhibiting impulses are not sent from the cortical bladder centre to prevent completion of the sacral reflex arc, and the bladder begins to contract before micturition is voluntarily initiated (Figure 2.4). This will usually cause symptoms of frequency, urgency, urge incontinence, and possibly nocturia or even nocturnal enuresis.

The unstable bladder, contracting uninhibitedly outside voluntary control, may be caused by an upper motor neurone lesion (e.g. a cerebrovascular accident) affecting the cortical micturition centre. Often sensation is left intact – the person appreciates the need to pass urine, but cannot delay this until the lavatory is reached. Sometimes urgency is total – precipitant micturition occurs simultaneously with sensation. At other times it may be less severe, with a diminished warning between sensation and capacity, but may still result in incontinence if the lavatory is not reached in time. It is possible also that general age-changes in the brain cause most very elderly people to have some degree of bladder instability (see Chapter 8).

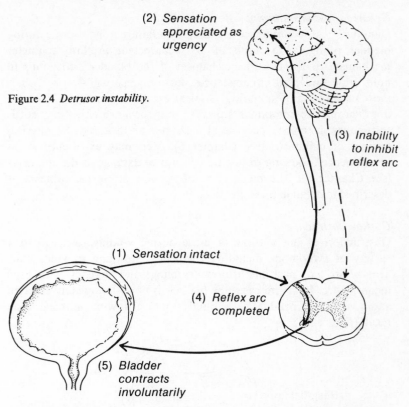

(2) *Sensation appreciated as urgency*

Figure 2.4 *Detrusor instability.*

(3) *Inability to inhibit reflex arc*

(1) *Sensation intact*

(4) *Reflex arc completed*

(5) *Bladder contracts involuntarily*

Many people with an unstable bladder have no obvious neurological lesion to explain their inability to inhibit bladder contractions. This includes most lifelong nocturnal enuretics (bedwetters) and other people without overt neuropathy. The condition often presents in the second, third or fourth decade of life with no obvious preceding cause. It is then called 'idiopathic detrusor instability', causing exactly the same symptoms as the unstable bladder occurring secondarily to an upper motor neurone lesion. In children, detrusor instability predominantly affects boys; in young adults it is commoner in women. Some workers have postulated a psychosomatic causation, others that the bladder control centre in the brain is congenitally malformed. Learning theorists have suggested it might be caused by a failure ever to learn effective subconscious bladder control. Minimal neurological or neurochemical imbalances have also been suggested. None of these explanations has been conclusively proven, so the condition, for the present, remains 'idiopathic'.

Genuine stress incontinence

Genuine stress incontinence is caused by a failure to hold urine during bladder filling, as a result of an incompetent urethral sphincter mechanism. If the closure mechanism of the bladder outlet fails to hold urine under all circumstances, incontinence will occur. This is most usually manifest during physical exertion or stress. (The term does *not* refer to emotional 'stress'.) It may occur in either sex, but is commoner in women because of a shorter urethra and the physical trauma of childbirth (see Chapter 6). Men may experience stress incontinence following traumatic or surgical damage to the sphincter (see Chapter 7). The mechanism of genuine stress incontinence is described in detail in these chapters.

Outflow obstruction

Obstruction of the outflow of urine during voiding can lead to a variety of symptoms, including frequency, straining to void, poor urinary stream, post-micturition dribbling, and urgency with urge incontinence. In severe cases the bladder is never completely emptied and a volume of residual urine builds up. Overflow incontinence may result (Figure 2.5).

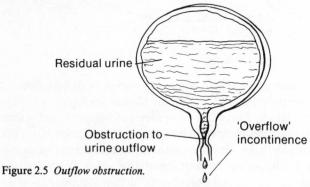

Residual urine

Obstruction to urine outflow

'Overflow' incontinence

Figure 2.5 *Outflow obstruction.*

This is most commonly associated with prostatic hypertrophy in older men (see Chapter 7). It may also occur in either sex because of urethral stenosis or stricture (possibly following instrumentation or infection of the urethra). Alternatively, a neurological lesion may prevent co-ordinated relaxation of the urethra during voiding, even in the absence of an actual anatomical obstruction to the outflow of urine ('detrusor-sphincter dyssynergia'). The urethra is in spasm and acts as an obstruction to the passage of urine (see Chapter 10).

The detrusor muscle of an obstructed bladder may become very powerful and hypertrophied, in an attempt to overcome the high outflow resistance. In some instances secondary detrusor instability may develop. If the obstruction is long-standing the bladder may eventually 'decompensate' – give up the unequal struggle to empty, and become atonic.

Atonic bladder
The atonic bladder is one which does not produce a proper voiding contraction for micturition. Emptying only occurs with abdominal effort or manual expression, and a large residual volume builds up. Sensation may or may not be present. Frequency will be common if sensation is present, as only a small proportion of bladder volume is utilised (Figure 2.6). Sensation is often diminished and the residual urine volume may reach considerable amounts (500–2000ml). Over-flow incontinence will often occur.

Atony is usually caused by damage to the peripheral nerves of the bladder (e.g. in diabetes), or by damage to the lower spinal cord or feedback loops to the brain stem (see Chapter 10).

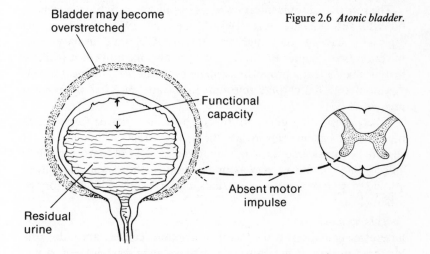

Bladder may become overstretched

Figure 2.6 *Atonic bladder.*

Functional capacity

Absent motor impulse

Residual urine

These four types of bladder dysfunction are very different in their mechanism of causing urinary incontinence. It is vital to distinguish between them because, as will be seen, the treatments are also very different. It is possible to have more than one of these problems at the same time, and for the elderly especially, multiple pathology is common.

FACTORS DIRECTLY INFLUENCING BLADDER FUNCTION

Some problems directly affect and upset the normal function of the bladder. Any of these factors, if severe enough, could cause incontinence even in someone with a normal bladder. More often they combine with one of the above bladder dysfunctions and lead to incontinence.

Urinary tract infection

An acute urinary tract infection (UTI) can cause transient incontinence even in a fit, healthy young person who normally has no bladder problems. Acute frequency and urgency with disturbed sensation and pain can cause inability to get to the lavatory in time, or to tell when incontinence is occurring. If an underlying bladder dysfunction is also present, an acute UTI is very likely to cause incontinence. Infection especially aggravates an unstable bladder and may increase the number and frequency of uninhibited contractions. The presence of residual urine in the bladder will predispose to an infection, which will be difficult to eradicate. The presence of incontinence may in turn increase the risks of acquiring UTI, especially in women wearing pads.

The role that chronic infection plays in causing incontinence is more doubtful (Brocklehurst et al., 1968; Milne et al., 1972). Elderly people especially have a very high prevalence of chronic urinary tract infection (see Chapter 8). Since many are also incontinent it is likely just by chance that a proportion will be both infected and incontinent. A causal role for chronic infection in incontinence has never been proven.

When considering infection, tuberculosis must not be forgotten as the tubercle bacillus can invade the urinary tract. Although rare, it should be considered as a potential cause of symptoms, especially among those living in very poor conditions, those who have lived abroad or who are recent immigrants, and in people with a history of tuberculosis.

Faecal impaction

Severe constipation with faecal impaction considerably disturbs bladder function. It may affect the bladder in several different ways. Sometimes the faeces in the rectum form a physical outflow obstruction to urine (Figure 2.7) by pressing on the bladder, urethra, and local nerves, thus leading to retention with overflow of urine. Direct pressure will also aggravate an unstable bladder. In other cases the impaction, by stretching the pelvic floor and inhibiting pelvic-floor contractions, leads to stress incontinence.

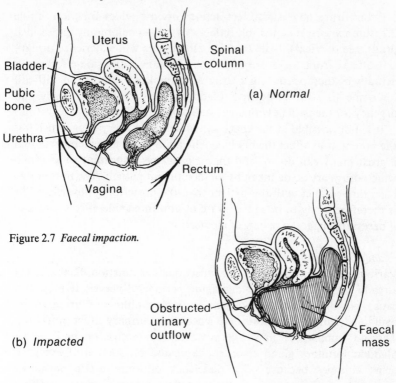

Figure 2.7 *Faecal impaction.*

Faecal impaction can also cause the sufferer to feel unwell, lethargic, and generally disinclined to activity. Many of the causes of faecal impaction (see Chapter 14) may also disturb continence, for example poor diet, low fluid intake, immobility, and a poor environment.

Drug therapy
Many drugs can disturb bladder function. The most obvious category is diuretics – a large, swift diuresis will give most people frequency and urgency. If the bladder is unstable it may not be able to cope with a sudden influx of urine, and urge incontinence may result. Sedation may either directly affect bladder function (e.g. diazepam may lower urethral resistance), or make the individual much less responsive to signals from the bladder and so fail to maintain continence. (For example, a person with an unstable bladder may find that night sedation means a good night's sleep and a wet bed, when without medication he is woken several times to pass urine.)

Other drugs have side-effect actions upon bladder function. Table 2.2 summarises the possible effects of some commonly prescribed drugs (see overleaf). Note that not all patients will experience urinary side-effects from these drugs. In some instances the side-effects may actually be therapeutic (e.g. a drug which makes voiding more difficult for someone with a 'normal' bladder may decrease frequency and urgency for the patient with an unstable bladder).

It is not possible in the space available to list every drug which has the potential to affect the bladder. The main point to remember is that a great many can do so, and that it is always important to ascertain which drugs are being taken by an incontinent patient. The nurse often has more contact with the patient than the prescribing physician. She is therefore likely to be more aware of unwanted side-effects, and can if necessary suggest a review of medication.

Endocrine disorders

Various endocrine disorders may upset bladder function. Diabetes has already been mentioned as damaging peripheral nerves. It may also cause polydipsia with a consequent large volume of urine to be contained, and glycosuria may encourage urinary tract infection. Thyroid imbalances may aggravate an overactive or underactive bladder. Pituitary gland disorders can cause production of excessive urine volumes because of a deficiency of anti-diuretic hormone. Oestrogen deficiency in post-menopausal women causes atrophic changes in the vagina and urethra, and will worsen both stress incontinence and an unstable bladder (see Chapter 8).

Miscellaneous bladder pathology

Several different bladder pathologies may cause incontinence by disrupting normal functioning. A neoplasm, whether benign or malignant, or a stone in the bladder may occasionally present with incontinence as a symptom. These are rare causes of incontinence.

FACTORS AFFECTING ABILITY TO COPE WITH THE BLADDER

Many people have one or more of the conditions outlined above without actually wetting themselves. People with an unstable bladder, a urinary tract infection, or who are taking diuretics often learn to prevent incontinence. They achieve this by visiting the lavatory at every available opportunity, never moving too far from a lavatory, or keeping a receptacle near at hand, such as a commode by the bed or a bucket under the sink, in case of being 'caught short'. They will only go shopping in a centre where they know all the lavatories, and the first thing they do on any outing (if they will go on one) is ascertain the quickest route to the nearest lavatory. Some isolate themselves completely and refuse to go out or mix socially. Younger people with an unstable bladder are often not incontinent simply because they are agile enough to respond quickly to urgency. Many people with a tendency to stress incontinence avoid leakage by avoiding physical exertion – they stop playing sport, do not go shopping if heavy weights may have to be carried, refuse to dance, and try not to laugh when out. When they have a cough they are more likely to stay at home in order to avoid potential embarrassment. People with difficulties in bladder emptying may spend excessive time in the lavatory trying to strain until the bladder is empty. Many incontinent people restrict fluid intake, often completely, in an attempt to prevent incontinence (see also pages 73–74).

Often it takes something else in addition to the underlying bladder problem to 'tip the balance' and produce incontinence. This is especially true for some of the elderly and disabled who are delicately balanced between continence and incontinence – a balance which can easily be tipped either way.

Any one of the following factors is in some cases sufficient reason alone for incontinence. More often they combine with an actual bladder problem to produce incontinence.

Immobility
To be able to pass urine in the 'correct' place you have to be able to get there. Anything which impedes access is likely to induce incontinence. Immobility may be the result of the gradual worsening of a chronic condition, such as arthritis, multiple sclerosis, or Parkinson's disease, until eventually the individual is simply unable to get to the lavatory in time. Or it may be acute: an accident or illness which suddenly renders a person immobile may be the start of his failure to control the bladder.

The importance of immobility is closely related to the degree of urgency experienced. If it takes longer to get to the lavatory or obtain an alternative receptacle (such as a bedpan) than the person can hold on, incontinence is the inevitable result. A very disabled person may become incontinent simply because he cannot get to or onto a lavatory, or because no help is at hand.

21

Table 2.2: Possible Side-effects Of Commonly Prescribed Drugs Upon Bladder Function

Drug	Main Uses	Action upon Urinary Tract	Possible Effect on Continence
Phenothiazines e.g. chlorpromazine	Neuroleptic Sedative Psychosis Anti-emetic	Relaxes smooth muscle (e.g. detrusor muscle)	Voiding difficulties and retention
Levodopa	Anti-Parkinsonian	Relaxes smooth muscle (e.g. detrusor muscle)	Voiding difficulties and retention
Propantheline	Peptic ulcer Pancreatitis	Relaxes smooth muscle (e.g. detrusor muscle)	Voiding difficulties and retention
Hydralazine	Anti-hypertensive	Relaxes smooth muscle (e.g. detrusor muscle)	Voiding difficulties and retention
Salbutamol	Bronchospasm of asthma or bronchitis	Increases smooth muscle tone in outflow tract	Voiding difficulties and retention (may relieve stress incontinence)
Phenylpropanolamine	Nasal decongestant	Increases smooth muscle tone in outflow tract	Voiding difficulties and retention (may relieve stress incontinence)
Propanolol	Anti-hypertensive	Increases smooth muscle tone in outflow tract	Voiding difficulties and retention (may relieve stress incontinence)

Drug	Main Uses	Action upon Urinary Tract	Possible Effect on Continence
Ergotamine	Migraine	Increases smooth muscle tone in outflow tract	Voiding difficulties and retention (may relieve stress incontinence)
Methyldopa	Anti-hypertensive	Decreases smooth muscle tone in outflow tract	Stress incontinence
Digoxin	Cardiac arrhythmias Congestive heart failure	Increased detrusor muscle tone	Increased bladder pressure, decreased capacity
Amitriptyline Imipramine	Anti-depressant	Anticholinergic	Voiding difficulties and retention (may relieve detrusor instability)

Note: Not all patients taking these drugs will experience urinary tract symptoms.

23

Linked closely with mobility are factors such as manual dexterity, eyesight, condition of the feet (and shoes), and suitability of clothing. (See Chapter 9 for a discussion of incontinence and the physically disabled.)

Environment

The physical design and layout of surroundings may or may not be ideal for easy continence. The situation of the lavatory, ease of access, and number of other people who share it (and might be using it) are important. In public places, including hospitals, many lavatories are considerable distances from main areas, and may be poorly marked and difficult to use if a person is disabled in any way. At home, there may be stairs to negotiate or the lavatory may be outside the house.

The social environment is also important. In some situations incontinence becomes the norm (especially in long-stay institutions), and the social pressure to be continent disappears. In a socially impoverished atmosphere people may lose their grip on reality and exhibit disordered behaviours, including incontinence. At home the isolated incontinent person may lose all motivation to try to maintain continence. The well-supported person with a good social network who is seen as a valid and useful member of the community (and sees himself as such) is most likely to make every effort to avoid incontinence and to seek help early if it does occur.

Mental function

People with lowered mental capabilities, whether because of mental handicap, confusion, or dementia, may not recognise the social need for continence or what is considered acceptable behaviour. This is seldom a sufficient reason on its own to explain incontinence. Many of them will also have an underlying bladder disorder (see above). The majority of people with disordered mental function are capable of continence with appropriate management (see Chapters 8 and 12), except possibly in cases of profound handicap or very advanced dementia. However, the confused elderly are very easily disorientated, and many who can cope well in their own surroundings cannot manage in a strange environment. Flexibility of reaction may be lost, and incontinence results.

Emotions

The bladder has been said to be a sensitive emotional barometer, and many people find their bladder function upset when they are upset – witness the queues for the lavatory outside an examination or interview room. The causal relationship of emotional problems to incontinence is unclear. There can be little doubt that many incontinent people appear depressed or anxious – but whether this is a cause or an outcome of incontinence is not yet known.

Incontinence may also be associated with emotional regression under stress, and in rare situations may be a symptom of protest or despair at an unacceptable life situation. Onset of incontinence may follow a traumatic life-event, such as bereavement. It may also be used as manipulative or 'attention-seeking' behaviour by a few patients. As mentioned above, some clinicians believe that idiopathic detrusor instability is psychosomatic in origin (although the evidence for this is inconclusive).

Carers

Those who are dependent upon other people to some degree for their continence are 'at risk' of becoming incontinent unless those carers, whether relatives, nurses, or others, are sensitive to their needs and orientated towards the promotion of continence. If the attitude of the carer is to expect and accept incontinence in the dependant, incontinence becomes much more likely.

In some instances, carers can actually promote incontinence by making it easier to be wet than dry. An individual may find that it is much less bother for carers to come and change a pad at intervals than to struggle to get to the lavatory. If incontinence seems to be the expected norm, and if it is rewarded by attention and physical and social contact, it may soon become established behaviour.

These and many other potential 'causes' of incontinence are dealt with in greater depth in the relevant chapters of this book. Any combination of problems is possible. Young, otherwise fit, incontinent people tend to have just one single bladder dysfunction underlying their symptom. Older and disabled people tend to have complex problems with many different factors combining to render them incontinent. The multiplicity of possible causes emphasises the importance of seeing incontinence as a symptom, the causes of which must be investigated and diagnosed accurately if treatment is to stand a chance of success. It should never simply be accepted as an inevitable consequence of ageing, disease, or disability. Often the assumed 'cause' is only part of the story. Today it is possible to modify most of the underlying bladder dysfunctions and in many cases to remedy them completely.

Most of the factors in the two categories discussed on pages 18–25 are also amenable to treatment.

There is no incontinent person for whom it is pointless to enquire 'Why?'. There must always be a cause; incontinence does not just happen. If nurses can keep that question – WHY? – in the forefront of their thinking when caring for incontinent people, many who are currently suffering from this symptom will stand a good chance of regaining continence.

REFERENCES AND FURTHER READING

Brocklehurst, J. C., Dillane, J. B., Griffiths, L., Fry, J., 1968. 'The prevalence and symptomatology of urinary tract infection in an aged population'. *Gerontologica Clinica*, 10, 242–253.

Milne, J. S., Williamson, J., Maule, M. M., Wallace, E. T., 1972. 'Urinary symptoms in older people'. *Modern Geriatrics*, 5, 198–212.

(See Appendix 3 for general reviews of the causes of incontinence.)

Chapter 3

Assessment and Investigation of Urinary Incontinence

Several different professionals may be involved in assessing and managing the incontinent patient. There can be little doubt that the team approach offers the optimum help for many patients, and the contribution of various paramedical personnel is dealt with in more detail in Chapter 4. This chapter concentrates on the nursing and medical aspects of assessment, but it should not be forgotten that under some circumstances a member of another profession may contribute part of the total picture.

Most commonly, the individual presenting for help with incontinence will be assessed and investigated by a nurse or doctor. Ideally a joint nursing and medical assessment should be made. Both professions have a valuable contribution to make in forming a comprehensive picture of why incontinence is occurring and how it is affecting the patient. However, we do not live in an ideal world and often nursing and medical assessments are made independently, with little liaison. Indeed, in many cases one or the other assessment is omitted completely. This chapter describes a comprehensive assessment, without specifying who should do what – this will often be a matter for local time, interest and expertise to determine. Nurses can do much of this assessment alone, but without medical support and interest the patient will not obtain the most accurate diagnosis possible.

PRESENTATION

The first bridge to be crossed in assessing incontinence is finding out who has the problem. (This may sound ridiculous to a nurse working in a long-stay unit where the problem is only too obvious and pervasive.) The vast majority of incontinent people live outside institutional settings and only rarely come into contact with the health

27

service. Many people hide their incontinence because of embarrassment or guilt, or accept it without question as an inevitable concomitant of age or disability. Not many people would wish to admit to a friend, neighbour, or relative that they were incontinent – it must be one of the least acceptable symptoms as a subject for conversation. Many others feel that as it is not 'serious' (i.e. life-threatening), it is not worth bothering their busy and overworked general practitioner with it. Some are too shy to discuss the topic with a doctor of the opposite sex. Even when a nurse is involved in a patient's care (whether inpatient or outpatient), the subject is seldom brought up.

Once incontinence is admitted, all too often the sufferer is met by a nurse or doctor who accepts it as a chronic untreatable condition. 'What do you expect at your age?' is not an uncommon remark, or 'You'll have to learn to live with it'. Sometimes this may be because of lack of knowledge: the nurse or doctor genuinely does not realise how much can be done to relieve it or else feels inadequate or hopeless. Acceptance may be compounded by embarrassment and the inability to talk easily about such problems. If the professional is embarrassed the patient will often pick this up and avoid further discussion of the topic. Often incontinence will have been mentioned during the course of a consultation or hospitalisation for another problem, and there is a temptation to revert to a 'safer' topic.

Starting to talk about incontinence can be difficult, because the sufferer has an inadequate vocabulary and does not know what terms to use. The word 'incontinent' is usually avoided or else used to denote total lack of control (see Chapter 8). Every care must be taken to establish a mutually understood terminology before the assessment is made. The patient who denies 'incontinence' may quite happily admit to an 'occasional leak'.

HISTORY

The first essential in assessing the nature and extent of incontinence is to take an accurate and full history. It is vital that whoever is taking this history has a sound basic knowledge of the subject and knows what questions to ask, and why. Also, that he or she understands the significance of the answers and knows which leads should be followed up. This history is not gathered for its own sake, but as a tool to aid accurate diagnosis and to help in planning treatment and care. It also provides a baseline from which to monitor progress, and a point of reference for other workers.

Where possible, the information should be gathered in a relaxed, informal atmosphere, preferably in the patient's usual environment. Plenty of time should be allowed, as this will often be the first time the patient has discussed the problem with anyone, and a hurried consultation may result in missing the main point or the extent of the problem. Incontinent people usually take a while to feel comfortable and able to discuss their incontinence, especially with a stranger.

The patient will often be able to answer all the necessary questions himself. Where he cannot, for reasons of poor memory, communication difficulties, or mental impairment, other sources of information should be used – medical records, talking to relatives or carers, and observation of the patient interacting with his surroundings. When the patient is mentally alert his permission should be sought before talking to relatives, as he may have gone to great lengths to disguise the problem, and may not wish others to know about it.

Much of this information would be gathered routinely in a nursing process assessment and would not need to be repeated as a separate 'incontinence assessment' (Norton, 1980).

CHECKLIST

Figure 3.1 (overleaf) gives an example of an assessment checklist which may be used as an aide-memoire when taking an incontinence history (Norton, 1984). It is not intended to be used inflexibly or administered as a questionnaire, but merely to ensure that all relevant areas are covered and that accurate and complete records are kept in a systematic fashion. Some questions require simply a 'yes/no' answer; others will require elaboration. Not all questions are likely to be relevant to every incontinent person. It has been found to be a useful tool for assessing both inpatients and outpatients. For some people a much more detailed history of specific aspects may be required (for instance, behavioural assessment for the mentally handicapped – see Chapter 12). The assessor should be constantly aware of the relevance and implications of each question. These are now discussed in detail.

Main complaint

It is important to note at the outset what the presenting problem is – either from the patient's perspective or that of the primary carer. An individual may have a great variety of different symptoms, of varying importance to him, and treatment or management should usually be directed in the first instance at solving those which are

Figure 3.1 *Incontinence Assessment Checklist*

Note: These headings will elicit the basic information needed for an assessment. The reader should construct a checklist using these headings (and any other found necessary and relevant for specific circumstances), leaving adequate space for filling in the answers and any comments.

Name: Date of Birth:

Address:

General Practitioner:

Assessed by: Date: Referred by:

1) MAIN COMPLAINT

2) URINARY SYMPTOMS

    Frequency: Nocturia (?Woken):

    Urgency: Average warning time: Urge incontinence:

    Stress incontinence: Passive incontinence:

    Nocturnal enuresis: Number of nights per week:

    Symptoms of voiding difficulty

    Hesitancy: Poor stream: Straining:

    Manual expression: Post-micturition dribble:

    Dysuria: Haematuria:

    Incontinence

    Onset – when?   Circumstances:

    Is incontinence improving/static/worsening?

    How often does incontinence occur?   How much is lost?

    Are aids or pads used?   type of aid:

        number per day: source of supply:

        are aids effective?   problems:

    Type and amount of fluid intake: Fluid restriction?

    Other urinary symptoms:

3) PAST MEDICAL HISTORY

    Previous illnesses/operations:

    Parity: Difficult deliveries?

    Current medication:

    Any previous treatment for incontinence?

4) BOWELS
   Usual bowel habit: Constipation?
   Laxatives or diet regulation used?
   Faecal incontinence?

5) MOBILITY
   Problems with mobility: Aids used?
   Needs assistance?   Who is available?
   Difficulties in transfer to/onto lavatory?   Comments:
   Foot problems: Manual dexterity:
   Clothing suitability: Eyesight:
   Observe self-toileting and comment on problems:
   Problems with personal hygiene:

6) PSYCHOLOGICAL STATE
   Attitude to incontinence:
   Anxiety?   Depression?
   Impaired mental abilities?

7) SOCIAL NETWORK
   Usual activities: Are these restricted by incontinence?
   Who does patient live with?   Who visits regularly?
   Relationship problems because of incontinence?
   Official services received:

8) ENVIRONMENT
   Lavatory facilities: Are urinals or commode used?
   Obstacles to using lavatory: Washing/laundry facilities:
   Comments on general physical and social environment:

9) RESULTS OF PHYSICAL EXAMINATION
   Skin problems: Prolapse (women):   Atrophic changes (women):
   Rectal examination: Post-micturition residual urine volume:
   MSSU/urine test result: Other findings:

10) RESULTS FROM CHART:

Summary of Problems:
Aims/Goals:
Planned Action: Review date:
Follow-up Notes:

causing the greatest problem. The patient may rate the severity of symptoms very differently from a nurse or doctor, so it is vital to ask his opinion: 'What, to you, is the *main* problem with your bladder/waterworks?' is a useful way of wording the question. The answer may be a common symptom – e.g. wetting on the way to the lavatory or wetting the bed – or it may be a highly idiosyncratic problem which is altering the sufferer's life-style – perhaps leaking when taking a swing at a golf ball, or during sexual intercourse.

Urinary symptoms

Urinary symptoms are notoriously unreliable indicators of underlying bladder dysfunction. It is impossible to make a totally reliable diagnosis of which bladder problem is present on history of symptoms alone. However, symptoms do give broad clues as to the likely diagnosis, and together with the rest of the history and a thorough examination, can predict the most likely dysfunction (such as detrusor instability, genuine stress incontinence, or retention with overflow incontinence). However, if surgery is contemplated, or if the presumptive diagnosis has not led to successful treatment, the bladder dysfunction needs to be confirmed by urodynamic tests (see pages 45–65). Patients who have a complex mixture of symptoms will often need urodynamic tests in the first instance.

Frequency of passing urine by day may be indicated by recording either the number of times urine is passed between rising and retiring, or the average time interval between toilet visits. Most people pass urine between three and six times per day (3- to 4-hourly). Seven or more times is usually classed as abnormally high frequency.

Nocturia means rising at night to pass urine. It is important to ascertain whether the patient is actually woken by bladder sensation, or whether he is already sleeping badly and simply getting up from boredom or to 'make sure' before getting back to sleep. Nocturia is a classic early symptom of prostatic enlargement in men. Some people always have to get up once in the night, although most rarely do so. Being woken twice or more is abnormal, although it becomes commonplace in extreme old age, probably because the normal diurnal variation in urinary excretion is lost.

If abnormally high frequency by day or by night is reported, the patient should be asked why this is so. Mostly it is because of feeling the desire to void. Occasionally, however, it is caused by old habits (for example, following childhood advice not to hold urine for too long). Because of an anxious or obsessional personality trait, the patient may feel a compulsion to use every available opportunity to empty the bladder. High frequency accompanied by discomfort may indicate a urinary tract infection or atrophic urethritis. Sometimes frequency is high simply because fluid intake is excessive (especially in women who have been advised to drink a lot following bouts of cystitis), or because diuretic medication is being taken.

A very low frequency of micturition might indicate a high-capacity bladder, dehydration, or retention of urine.

Excessive frequency is most commonly associated with detrusor instability – bladder contractions giving frequent sensations of the desire to void. It may also occur in genuine stress incontinence, because urine in an open bladder-neck makes the patient feel the need to empty the bladder. A patient with a large residual volume may pass urine very frequently because the functional capacity of the bladder (the actual volume available for filling and emptying) is considerably reduced.

Urgency is the symptom of having to hurry to pass urine. The warning time between the first sensation of bladder filling and an urgent need to empty the bladder is curtailed. There may only be ten minutes' warning instead of an hour or so, or the need can be so urgent that normal activities have to be interrupted and a lavatory found immediately. Sometimes precipitancy is present – the bladder starts to empty simultaneously with first bladder sensation, with no prior warning at all. If urgency is not responded to, or if the environment is unsuitable, *urge incontinence* may result. This is the symptom of not being able to get to or onto the lavatory in time. Again, this may be partial or complete, and will often depend on how fast the sufferer can move and how far it is to the nearest lavatory.

Urgency and urge incontinence are most commonly due to detrusor instability. However, they can also occur with most other bladder problems.

Stress incontinence is the symptom of leaking urine coincidentally with physical exertion (*not* emotional stress), such as coughing, laughing or lifting. It may be mild – occurring only on strenuous exercise. In severe cases the effort of rising from a chair or walking may cause incontinence.

Stress incontinence is usually associated with genuine stress incontinence, i.e. a weakness or incompetence of the urethral sphincter mechanism. It may also occur in people with an unstable bladder (for example, a cough may trigger a bladder contraction) or with overflow incontinence.

33

Passive incontinence is wetting at rest without any coincident activity or sensation. Typically the patient will complain of 'just finding myself wet' for no apparent reason. Most often the underlying bladder problem is retention with overflow.

Nocturnal enuresis is bedwetting while asleep. This must be distinguished from nocturia with urge incontinence, where the patient wakes but cannot get up in time. In people of all ages, from children to the very elderly, nocturnal enuresis is usually caused by detrusor instability.

Symptoms of *voiding difficulty* should be sought. Hesitancy is having to wait, once in position, for the flow of urine to start. Most men will know if their stream has diminished in force, but many women cannot answer this unless the problem is severe and urine dribbles out very slowly. Straining, having to use abdominal effort, or manual expression, may be necessary to empty the bladder. Post-micturition dribbling is a small, usually passive, leak of urine 'when you think you have finished', most usually when clothing has been replaced. It may indicate trapping of urine in the bulbar urethra in men (see Chapter 7), or a urethral diverticulum in women. Some people feel that they never completely empty the bladder but are unable to pass the rest, however much they try.

All these symptoms of a voiding difficulty may be caused by either an obstructed or atonic bladder.

Dysuria means pain or burning while actually passing urine. Usually this is caused by a urinary tract infection or atrophic urethritis.

Haematuria (blood in urine) is a serious sign and immediate medical investigation should ensue, because a bladder carcinoma may be present.

Questions must be asked about the *incontinence* itself. Too often it is just reported as a fact without any further elaboration. The nurse should enquire: when did it start, and were there any specific circumstances associated with the onset of symptoms? Is the condition static, or is it worsening or improving? Does it vary, and under what circumstances is it worse or better? How often does incontinence occur? The actual volume of leakage is important as it may determine the most appropriate management. This can be difficult to estimate, especially as a little urine can spread a long way. A simple indication of the scale of the problem will suffice for most assessments, e.g. 'a few drops', 'wet pants', 'a moderate amount', 'soaked'. The only way to gauge incontinence accurately is by weighing pads before and after use, but this is seldom necessary except for research purposes.

Individual perceptions and tolerances of incontinence vary greatly.

What is a problem to one person will be classed as normal for another. Some fastidious people are very disturbed by a few drops leaking once per month. Others seem unconcerned by incontinence occurring several times a day. Volume and frequency of loss are not directly related to the amount of distress caused. Current symptoms will be interpreted according to pre-morbid bladder habits and expectations.

Aids, pads, or appliances may be already used. If so, it should be noted how many are used. Pad usage is not a reliable indicator of incontinence volume – many people change pads routinely rather than waiting until they are soaked to capacity. Often the aid will not be the ideal one and any problems (e.g. leakage, discomfort, odour) should be noted, together with source (e.g. self-purchase, district nurse, or prescription), and any problem with supply.

Fluid restriction is used by many incontinent people in an attempt to control their problem. Some find that certain types of fluid particularly upset the bladder – tea, coffee, and alcohol being the most common offenders. One of the most useful ways of determining the pattern of continence and incontinence is by using a chart (see page 41).

Past medical history

Note should be made of any past medical history that could influence either bladder function or the ability to cope with it. An obstetric history should record the number of babies, type of delivery, any particular difficulties, or heavy babies. A history of gynaecological, urological or neurological disease or surgery may be relevant, as may psychiatric problems or mental handicap. Current medical problems and general state of health should be noted. Any drug therapy may be relevant because so many drugs have an effect upon bladder function (see Chapter 2).

Bowels

Careful inquiry is needed to elicit 'normal' bowel habit and any significant change which has occurred. Bowel function varies greatly (see Chapter 14) and care must be taken not to impose arbitrary criteria for disturbed function. 'Constipation' is related more to difficulty of passing motions and their consistency than to frequency of defaecation. Faecal incontinence should be specifically asked about since it is even more embarrassing than urinary incontinence, and many people who will discuss the latter are unwilling to volunteer the fact that they also suffer soiling.

Mobility

Information about mobility problems will be gathered both by interview and direct observation. Mobility may be impaired directly or because movement is painful, or the patient may be unsteady and afraid to move. Any mobility aids (stick, frame, wheelchair) should be inspected for suitability and ease of use in the context of usual surroundings – e.g., is the lavatory space adequate to accommodate the walking frame? For the physically disabled, speed of mobility should be assessed in conjunction with the degree of urgency and the availability of help at the times it is needed. Ability to transfer safely from bed to commode or from wheelchair to lavatory will depend both on physical abilities and on the suitability of equipment design. On occasion, mobility is restricted by something as simple as inappropriate footwear (such as sloppy slippers which are difficult to walk in), unsafe loose mats, or by painful toenails which a visit to the chiropodist could remedy.

Manual dexterity: Linked closely to mobility is the degree of manual dexterity. It is useless being able to get to the lavatory in time if, once there, pants cannot be removed or skirts pulled up out of the way. It is very nearly as inconvenient to be incontinent in the lavatory as it is to be so on the way there. The best way to assess manual abilities is to watch the patient toilet himself, if this is thought to be a problem. The temptation may be great to offer assistance but this should be resisted during assessment.

Sometimes the problem is that an incontinence pad is not completely removed and urine is accidentally passed onto it while the patient is on the lavatory. The style of clothing may make dexterity problems worse: many layers of tight clothing, or buttons and stiff zips, may be the deciding factor between continence and incontinence, especially for those with urgency. Some people have praxis disorders – their manual abilities are disorientated in space so that they lose the ability to manipulate objects accurately. They are likely to make mistakes, like replacing a pad with the wrong side to the body, or be unable to dress and undress correctly.

Eyesight is also relevant here. Impaired vision can limit ability to get to or onto the lavatory, or lead to the incomplete removal of clothing or to missing a hand-held urinal. This can be a particular problem for men using a bottle.

Personal hygiene: Physical disabilities may impair the patient's ability to cope well with personal hygiene. Effective bathing or washing depends on having reasonable use of the hands and arms in particular. Even using lavatory paper may become impossible for those with arthritic shoulders or a weak grasp. Good personal hygiene is very important in preventing skin problems and odour. Even slight incontinence can render the person uriniferous and sore if hygiene is poor. Occasionally the incontinent person seems totally unconcerned about hygiene, and unaware of how far outside accepted social standards he has become. More often the converse is true – the incontinent person becomes overly obsessed by a fear of smelling. For most people this is an unrealistic and unnecessary fear, since with reasonable care odour need not arise.

Psychological state
Physical factors alone will not give a full picture of the individual and his incontinence.

The patient's attitude to incontinence will affect the treatment options. Most incontinent people are understandably distressed by their incontinence and are more than anxious to try anything that might help. Some people seem apathetic – they are convinced it is irreversible and think they have learned to accept it. This has often been reinforced by professional advice. Others deny the problem, even in the face of obvious evidence to the contrary. It may be denied because of shame, and the individual may blame someone or something else for a puddle (e.g. the cat, or a spilled flower vase). A few seem to deny incontinence even to themselves. It may be so unacceptable to them to admit the problem that they are genuinely unaware of it. This reflects a grave psychological conflict between reality and the individual's self-image. It may take a long time and much effort to gain the patient's confidence and bolster up his self-concept before he can admit the problem. A few never do – helping them becomes very difficult as any treatment or aids are rejected as unnecessary.

Some incontinent people appear very anxious or depressed. This may even be severe enough to constitute a psychiatric illness. Anxiety and depression might not only be a reaction to incontinence, but may also contribute to causing incontinence. Once the two problems co-exist it is not difficult to envisage how each might reinforce the other.

Those with impaired mental function, whether because of mental handicap, a confusional state or dementia, are less likely to be able to cope with the complex social requirements for continence. It may be useful to make a formal assessment of cognitive and social functioning (see Chapter 12 for a behavioural assessment of a mentally handicapped person). In some circumstances it may be appropriate to ask a psychologist or psychiatrist to contribute to the assessment of incontinence.

Social network
An individual's social contacts will often determine how well a problem is coped with. Many incontinent people deliberately isolate themselves and refuse to participate in former social activities. A note should be made of any curtailment of these that is occasioned by incontinence. If the patient lives with others, one should find out if the incontinence is affecting them as well, and what their attitude is to the problem. Stresses are often caused, whatever the age of the sufferer. Extra laundry, reluctance to go out, and the unpleasantness of incontinence can all put a strain on relationships, whether with child, spouse, parent, friend or landlady. At times the problem can become acute and be a factor in child abuse, matrimonial disharmony, or refusal to care any longer for an elderly relative. Sexual relationships are often disrupted because of incontinence during intercourse, or bedwetting. The whole family is often disrupted if one member is incontinent, whether because they feel unable to go away on holiday because a child wets the bed, or because they cannot go on outings because one member has to be continually stopping and looking for a lavatory, or because of a reluctance to invite relatives and friends in if heavy incontinence causes the house to smell.

Most incontinent people are not receiving any help from the health or social services. Assessment should be made of whether any services would be appropriate or, if they are being provided, whether they are the most appropriate (see Chapter 11). Once someone is receiving services their needs are often never re-assessed. Any change in circumstances may indicate the need for more, less, or different services.

Whether the sufferer is in institutional care or living at home, the social environment may be such as to promote continence or encourage incontinence. Assessment should include an impression of the prevailing atmosphere in which the individual is functioning and how this might influence continence.

Environment
The importance of the environment to the individual's ability to cope with bladder function has already been emphasised. Particular note should be made of lavatory facilities and any obstacles in reaching

them (e.g. stairs, long distances, cramped conditions, chairs or beds which are difficult to get out of). In institutions, good signposting and lighting may help the disorientated or visually handicapped. The lavatory itself may be the wrong height, unclean, or difficult to get onto. Privacy is important and too often neglected.

Does the person have access to good washing, laundry, and drying facilities? How are used aids to be disposed of? Unfortunately, many of the people liable to be incontinent are also likely to have the poorest facilities.

The extent to which incontinence is contained or is contaminating the environment should be noted. In extreme cases incontinence becomes the overwhelming factor in the environment, and is so poorly dealt with that total squalor results.

Results of physical examination

Ideally every incontinent person should have a full medical examination, including neurological, vaginal and rectal examination, and assessment of all major body systems as a screen for other health problems. In practice this ideal is not always attained. However, a nursing assessment should also include a basic examination of the patient. Careful observation will tell the nurse much about the general state of health, mobility, confusion, and mental state. Inspection of the genital area will reveal skin problems, an obvious vaginal prolapse, or atrophic changes in the vulva. A digital rectal examination will indicate if gross faecal impaction is present. Where stress incontinence is suspected it may be elicited with the patient standing with a full bladder and coughing vigorously.

A good case can be made for the measurement of residual urine volume after voiding to be included as a basic element of assessment. Too often significant voiding problems are overlooked, and a simple in-out catheter will alert the nurse or doctor to this possibility. In younger patients residual volume is usually nil immediately after micturition, although a volume up to 50ml is generally accepted as not being significant. In the older population (over 75 years) up to 100ml is considered to be within normal limits. The patient who has a larger residual volume should be investigated for a voiding problem.

A midstream or catheter specimen of urine should be collected for routine ward testing and microscopy, culture and sensitivity screening. Several different problems may be diagnosed, such as glycosuria (possible diabetes mellitus), high specific gravity (possible dehydration), or infection.

Results from charting

The chart is probably the single most useful nursing tool in assessing incontinence. At the same time it is often also the most misused. Charting is not an end in itself, but acts as a record to be interpreted in the light of all the other findings of the assessment, and as an aid in diagnosis and care planning. Charts are too often kept for long periods of time, even indefinitely, and either left on a clipboard at the foot of the patient's bed or filed in the back of notes, with totals columns carefully filled in, but with no action resulting from them.

The chart has two main uses: as a part of the baseline assessment of the individual's incontinence, and later as a record of progress during treatment, to monitor the effectiveness of therapy. Indeed, for bladder training programmes it forms the cornerstone of the regime (see Chapter 4). To be useful, a chart must be kept accurately – a seemingly obvious necessity that is often ignored. When a chart is being kept it is important that all staff know about it and that it is clear who is responsible for it. This must include night staff, domestic staff, visitors, and the patient himself. On a ward this is usually most reliably achieved where patient allocation is practised – each nurse knows whose chart she is responsible for on each shift. In many instances much more responsibility could be given to the patient to fill in his own chart – he is the only person present twenty-four hours a day – and it is beneficial to engage his interest in the problem at the outset. In the case of outpatients the patient or a relative will have to keep the chart, and many take a pride in keeping an accurate and neat chart for their doctor or nurse to examine, often doing it better than many nurses!

To be reliably accurate the chart should ideally be filled in as events occur (rather than at the end of the day from memory). The place where the chart is kept may influence the likelihood of this happening. While always remembering that it may cause embarrassment for a chart to be on public view, it is in some circumstances best to keep the chart in the lavatory, sluice, or with the patient (in a pocket or handbag). If the patient is in a dayroom with a nearby lavatory, a chart hanging on his bed or in the nurse's office, which may be a considerable distance away, is much more likely to be forgotten or else only filled in after a time lag.

Many different charts are available, some interchangeable, others with different functions. Before choosing a chart it is important to decide what information is needed. At its very simplest (Figure 3.2) a chart should show voidings and episodes of incontinence. This particular chart was designed to be easy to fill in and suitable for both inpatient and outpatient use. The less information that is requested, the greater the likelihood of it being kept accurately. With bold colouring and simple instructions most people (patients or nurses) are able to recognise easily what is expected and to fill it in accurately. Such a chart, kept for about one week, gives the nurse and patient a good baseline reading of the incontinence.

Figure 3.2 *Continence chart.*

Continence Chart

Week commencing _____ Name _____

Please tick in LEFT column each time urine is passed

Please tick in RIGHT column each time you are wet

	Monday	Tuesday	Wednesday	Thursday	Friday	Saturday	Sunday
6 am							
7 am							
8 am							
9 am							
10 am							
11 am							
12 pm							
1 pm							
2 pm							
3 pm							
4 pm							
5 pm							
6 pm							
7 pm							
8 pm							
9 pm							
10 pm							
11 pm							
12 am							
1 am							
2 am							
3 am							
4 am							
5 am							
Totals							

Special Instructions

For some purposes more information than this chart provides may be desirable. A frequency/volume chart will give an idea of functional bladder capacity, and this is often combined with an input estimation – a 'fluid balance chart'. Measuring input will highlight both polydipsia (excessive thirst – possibly a sign of metabolic disorder such as diabetes mellitus) and low fluid intake (possibly caused by fear of incontinence, which may eventually cause dehydration, constipation, electrolyte imbalance, and confusion, especially in an elderly patient). When interpreting the results, it should be noted whether the input was measured or just estimated.

Some charts do not specify times but are left blank, to be filled in as necessary. This means that times can be recorded more accurately than to the nearest hour. The assessment chart shown in Figure 3.3 also incorporates information about the patient's behaviour. This requires a nurse's signature – especially useful where patient allocation is not practised, since whoever supervised the episode can be easily identified. This chart is obviously designed for use by a nurse or carer, where the patient is incapable of self-care. It would reveal the patient's pattern of continence and incontinence, his ability to indicate needs, and the success of any toileting programme already being used. It is also useful in distinguishing between whether toileting was requested (i.e. patient-

CONTINENCE ASSESSMENT CHART

Name..

TOILETING REGIME
  − No
  ✓ Yes

Date	Time	Is patient incontinent of urine?	Did patient ask for toilet?	or	Routine toileting?	Did patient pass urine?	Signatures

Figure 3.3 *Continence assessment chart (courtesy of Longmore Hospital, Edinburgh).*

initiated) or nurse-initiated. If toileting does not result in urine being passed, this may mean either that it is being done at the wrong time, or that sensation is inaccurate (if the patient asked), or that, in the case of a demented patient, the realisation of what a lavatory is for has been lost. If a patient is toileted without result and is subsequently wet within a short period, this may indicate confusion about the social meaning of a toilet, or possibly that the patient was inhibited from emptying his bladder by lack of privacy, or by being rushed, and is suffering 'respite micturition' when relaxed back in the chair or bed.

Figure 3.4 (overleaf) shows a habit retraining chart which can also be used for baseline measurements (Clay, 1978). It presupposes regular checks (e.g. every two hours) on the state of the patient (this being recorded on the left of the hour line) and subsequent offering of toilet facilities and recording of the result on the right of the hour line. Some nurses find this complicated at first, but it gives a clear visual impression of any pattern and most people soon learn how to record accurately. Four coloured pens are needed.

Some charts use letters rather than ticks or dots as their symbols. This can increase the amount of information which can be gathered in the same space. However, it may also cause confusion if too many different letters are used, or if they are too similar and may be misread.

For some patients it may be useful to record events occurring simultaneously with incontinence – for example, a cough, or severe urgency. It may be useful to have an indication of how wet the patient was – 'incontinent' may mean anything from a few drops to a bladderful. This might be done by indicating when a pad was changed (but remembering this does not always necessarily mean that it was soaked), by indicating 'size of wet patch', or how far it spread (pants only, pad wet, clothes wet, leaked into environment). However, the only completely accurate assessment of volume would entail weighing pads, and this is seldom indicated.

When considering confused patients, it may be useful to record behavioural assessment information on the chart: what the patient was doing prior to the incontinence; what indication, if any, was given that incontinence had occurred (e.g. verbal or activity); and what were the subsequent results – how did staff/carers or others around react in response to incontinence? A record showing what happens when the patient voids continently and how he is responded to when dry would also be useful (see Chapter 8).

Usually an assessment chart will need to be kept for four to seven days in order to obtain an accurate picture of the current problem.

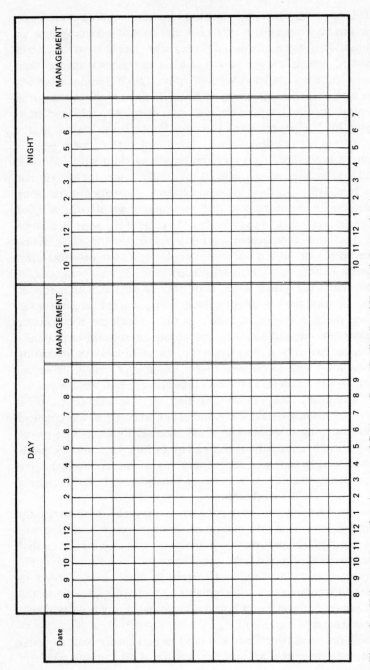

Figure 3.4 *Habit retraining chart (courtesy of Geriatric Dept., Dudley Road Hospital, Birmingham).* Key: (i) State of Patient: Dry – green dot; Incontinent of urine – red dot. (ii) Result of Toileting: Urine passed in toilet – blue dot; Urine not passed in toilet – yellow dot; Refused or absent – X in blue.

44

This will help to put the problem into perspective. Indeed, sometimes the mere act of charting reduces the incontinence – possibly by focussing the patient's or the staff's attention on the problem (those who were previously forgetful being more likely to remember to visit the toilet regularly). It also often happens that a problem which seemed random and out of control is in fact not so bad as was supposed, and the chart shows that the incontinence is reasonably predictable.

SUMMARY OF PROBLEMS

What conclusions may be drawn from the information gathered during this assessment? A detailed picture should have been built up of the individual as well as of the problems causing and caused by incontinence. Table 3.1 (see page 54) summarises the most common relationship of symptoms to medical problems, likely exacerbating factors, and underlying bladder dysfunction. However, it cannot be over-emphasised that many patients do not have a simple problem, and that any combination of factors may exist. This assessment should have enabled identification of the *most likely* bladder dysfunction, factors affecting bladder function, and factors affecting the individual's ability to cope with it. In the light of these findings, realistic aims or goals can be set for each individual and a plan of action formulated. A date should be set to review the outcome of this management.

Where symptoms are mixed or ambiguous, where surgery may be offered, or where treatment of presumed causes has not resulted in continence, further investigation by urodynamic studies may be indicated. While urodynamic studies are by no means essential for every incontinent patient, they are invaluable in contributing to a difficult or doubtful diagnosis. Conversely, urodynamics alone will often not be able to determine why a particular individual is incontinent. The results from such tests must be interpreted in the light of findings from the total assessment.

URODYNAMIC STUDIES

Urodynamics is the study of pressure and flow relationships in the lower urinary tract. Although such measurements have been made for decades, the science is still in its infancy. The clinical significance of many of the findings is open to debate, especially in the more sophisticated areas of investigation. This discussion is confined to the simpler and generally accepted findings from urodynamic studies. (For a more detailed discussion of techniques see Griffiths, 1980; Stanton, 1978 and 1984; Mandelstam, 1980.)

There are now over forty centres around the UK where urodynamics is available. The investigation department may be run variously by a urologist, gynaecologist, geriatrician, radiologist, or physicist, depending upon local interest and expertise. Often several of these specialists collaborate. Obviously, not every incontinent person is within easy reach of a urodynamic clinic and many have to travel considerable distances to reach one. In many instances the effort is well justified. It is to be hoped that urodynamic clinics will continue to spread so that eventually every District Health Authority will have at least one centre for urodynamic studies (recommendation of the Incontinence Action Group, 1983).

Three investigations form the basis of urodynamic studies: measurement of urinary flow rate, cystometry, and urethral pressure profile.

FLOW RATE

The rate of urinary flow during micturition can be measured simply and non-invasively by use of a flow meter (Figures 3.5 and 3.6). The rate at which urine is passed is measured either by a weight transducer under the receptacle or by a revolving disc inside the commode itself. A flow rate is expressed in millilitres of urine passed per second. The patient, whose bladder should be comfortably full, is asked to pass urine in privacy (women seated, men usually standing) into the flow meter. The flow rate is recorded on a chart which plots rate against time.

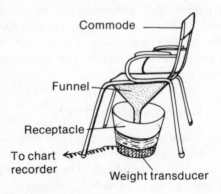

Figure 3.5 *Weight transducer flowmeter.*

46

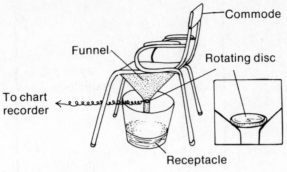

Figure 3.6 *Rotating disc flowmeter.*

Figure 3.7 shows a normal flow curve – the flow starts promptly, builds up to a good peak rapidly, and then drops again smoothly. When the volume of urine passed is over 200ml, a normal flow rate is at least 15ml per second. Figure 3.8 (overleaf) shows some typical abnormalities.

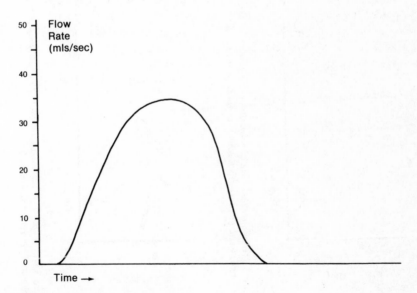

Figure 3.7 *Normal flow curve.*

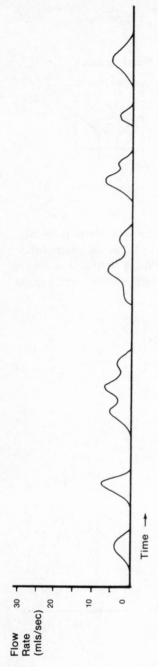

Figure 3.8 *Common flow-rate abnormalities. (a) Typical of an atonic bladder. Note the unsustained pattern of voiding. Bladder emptying is by abdominal effort, which cannot be prolonged for more than a few seconds.*

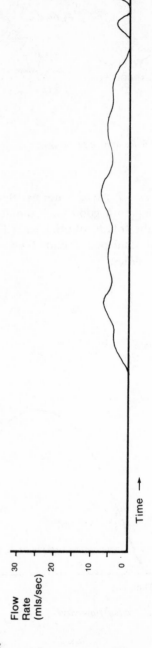

Figure 3.8(b) *Typical of outflow obstruction. Note the long period of hesitancy before flow commences and the protracted flow, which may be interrupted terminally.*

48

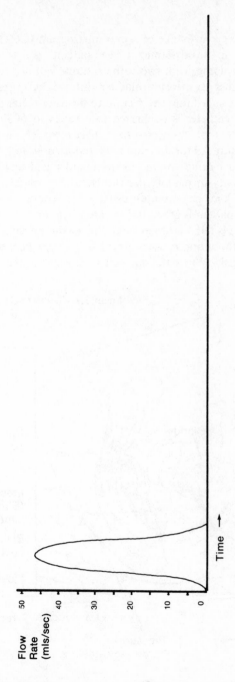

Figure 3.8(c) *Typical of sphincter incompetence. Note the high, precipitant flow rate, suggesting very low outflow resistance.*

CYSTOMETRY

Cystometry, or the performance of a cystometrogram (CMG), is the key investigation in urodynamics. The patient is catheterised, immediately after voiding, with two catheters: one will be used to fill the bladder, the other to measure bladder (intravesical) pressure. A catheter is also introduced into the rectum to measure rectal pressure. The bladder-filling catheter is connected to a reservoir of fluid. The two pressure catheters are connected to a chart recorder via pressure transducers (see Figure 3.9 for diagrammatic representation). A note is made of any residual urine volume in the bladder and any unusual difficulty or sensitivity in passing the catheters. The bladder is then filled rapidly (60–100ml per minute), usually with room-temperature normal saline. The patient is asked to indicate when the first sensation of the desire to void is felt, and then when the maximum capacity that can be tolerated without undue discomfort has been reached, trying all the while not to leak. When the subjective capacity is reached the

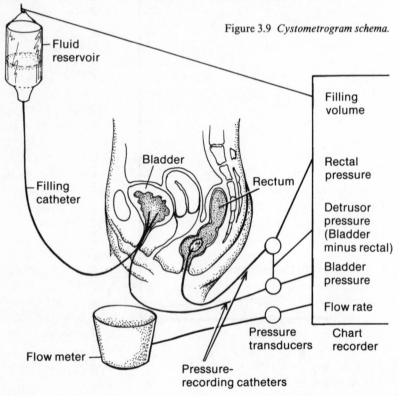

Figure 3.9 *Cystometrogram schema.*

filling catheter is removed, the patient is asked to stand up and cough vigorously. Various other 'provocative' tests may be tried, such as running a tap, drinking cold water, or jumping or walking on the spot. Any incontinence is noted. The patient is then instructed to void into a flow meter, as above. In midstream the patient is asked to attempt to interrupt the flow, and then void to completion.

The purpose of the rectal line is to monitor abdominal pressure. Because the bladder is an intra-abdominal organ the pressure inside it reflects both actual bladder activity and general abdominal-pressure changes. All movement and activities affect total bladder pressure, but these pressure changes are not necessarily the bladder itself doing anything. If bladder pressure alone were measured it would be very difficult to distinguish a bladder contraction from, say, the patient straining. The rectal pressure is measured to take account of these general abdominal-pressure changes, and the chart recorder subtracts rectal pressure from total bladder pressure to give a reading of bladder activity alone – detrusor pressure.

Figure 3.10 shows the trace from a normal cystometrogram. Residual urine should be zero. Pressure rise during filling of the bladder should be minimal – always below 15cm water pressure to be within normal limits. The bladder expands to accept urine without the intravesical pressure rising very much. First desire to void is usually felt at about half of capacity, and total comfortable volume is usually 400–600ml. Even at capacity the bladder should be stable and not contract. Vigorous coughing and provocative tests should not cause incontinence. When the patient is instructed to void, the bladder should contract smoothly (with a pressure around 30–40cm H_2O for women, 50–60cm H_2O for men), and the flow start very soon afterwards. The patient should be able to interrupt flow promptly, initially by closing the sphincter and then by inhibiting the contraction, and be able to re-start at will. The bladder should empty completely.

It is usually possible to conduct a cystometrogram with minimal embarrassment and discomfort to the patient. Great care should be taken to explain the procedure fully, both before the test and while it is in progress. Every effort should be made to maintain maximum privacy under the circumstances. Where feasible it is usually preferable that someone of the same sex as the patient should perform the catheterisation and supervise the procedure. If the patient is very anxious or frightened the results of the tests are often difficult to interpret, as it may be difficult to distinguish between inhibited voiding and a genuine voiding difficulty.

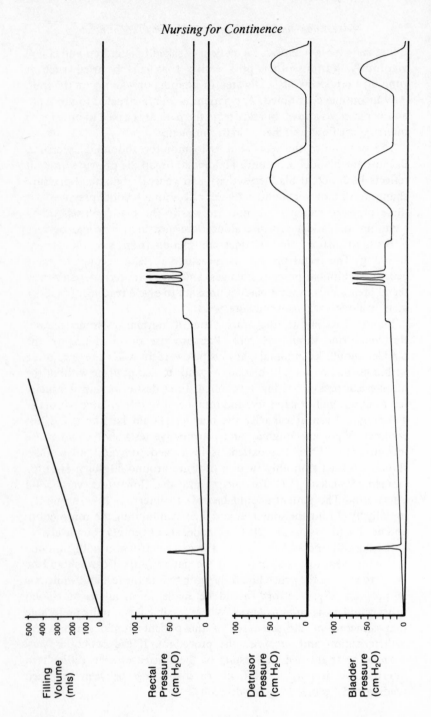

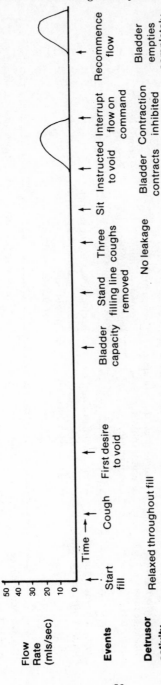

Figure 3.10 *Normal cystometrogram trace.*

Table 3.1: Relationship of Symptoms to Bladder Dysfunction
(Note — This Table gives broad generalisations only)

Patient's main symptoms	Most likely bladder dysfunction	Commonly associated medical problems	Factors likely to exacerbate symptoms
Urgency, urge incontinence Frequency Nocturia Nocturnal enuresis	Detrusor instability	Upper motor neurone lesion, e.g. CVA, multiple sclerosis, dementia; or may be 'idiopathic'	Immobility or other physical disabilities Poorly designed environment Anxiety
'Stress' incontinence (leakage upon physical exertion)	Genuine stress incontinence (urethral sphincter incompetence)	Vaginal prolapse Atrophic vaginitis Past obstetric difficulties Post-prostatectomy	Chronic cough Obesity
Dribbling incontinence and/or difficulty voiding	Atonic bladder or outflow obstruction leading to retention with overflow	Atonic: lower motor neurone lesion, e.g. diabetic neuropathy Spinal injury Obstructed: prostatic hypertrophy	Faecal impaction
Passive incontinence without warning or apparent reason	Any of above, or no specific bladder dysfunction	Often mental impairment, e.g. dementia, confusion, mental handicap	Disorientation, strange surroundings Physical handicaps Carers unaware of individual's needs Institutionalisation or poor motivation

Figure 3.11 (pp. 56–65) shows several of the most common abnormalities to be diagnosed by CMG. Figure 3.11(a) shows an unstable bladder or detrusor instability. The patient is unable to inhibit contractions during filling, and capacity is usually lowered. Incontinence may occur if contractions are high enough. Figure 3.11(b) shows genuine stress incontinence – essentially normal bladder function with incontinence during coughing and usually a high flow rate, low voiding pressure, and often impaired ability to interrupt flow. Figure 3.11(c) shows instability mimicking stress incontinence. This is an easily missed diagnosis – incontinence does occur with effort but because the cough triggers a contraction, and not because the sphincter is incompetent. Figure 3.11(d) shows an atonic bladder with a large residual capacity, delayed or absent sensation, and no voiding contraction – any voiding which occurs is achieved by abdominal effort. Figure 3.11(e) shows outflow obstruction. Voiding pressure is high in an attempt to overcome outflow resistance but the resultant flow is poor.

Thus all those physiological bladder dysfunctions described in Chapter 2 can be accurately differentiated by cystometrogram.

Added sophistication can be gained by performing cystometry under X-ray control (videocystourethrography). The bladder is filled with X-ray contrast instead of saline, and may be visualised during filling, coughing, and voiding. This is especially useful in distinguishing bladder-neck abnormalities and locating the site of an obstruction. Bladder diverticula, reflux of urine into the ureters, and various other abnormalities may be revealed.

URETHRAL PRESSURE PROFILE

Intra-urethral pressure can be measured by using either a water-filled or a microtransducer catheter, which is withdrawn slowly along the urethra with the patient in a supine position. A recording is obtained of urethral pressure from the bladder neck to the external meatus. At present this investigation is mostly used as a research tool, and its clinical relevance has yet to be firmly established.

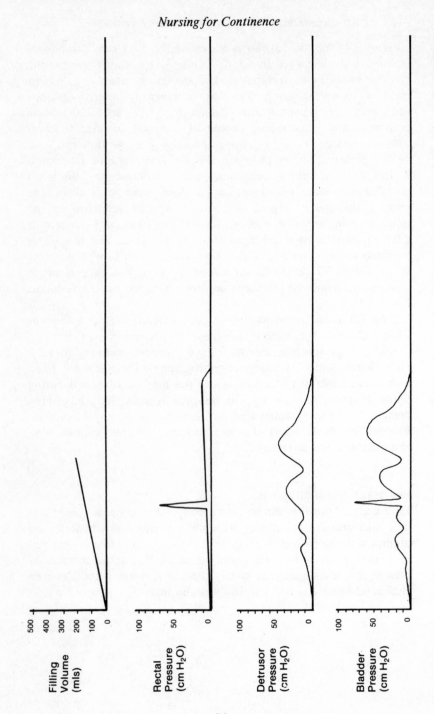

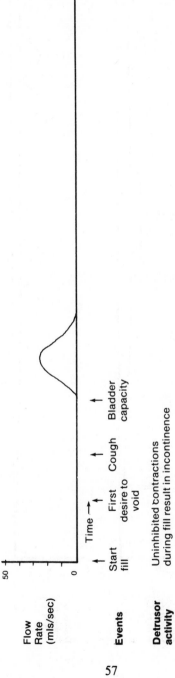

Figure 3.11 *Cystometrogram traces showing abnormalities.* (a) *Detrusor instability.*

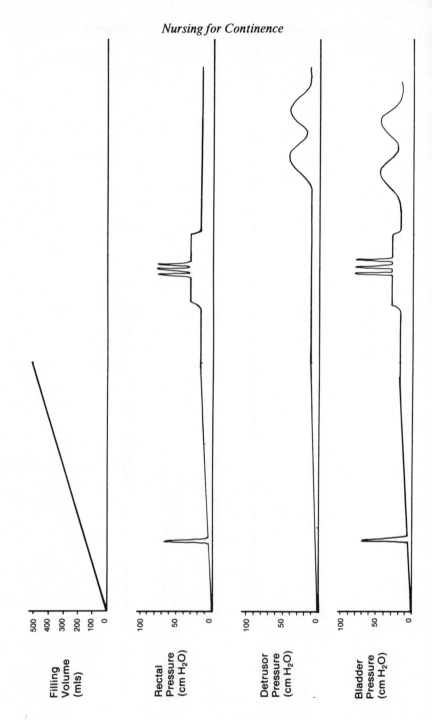

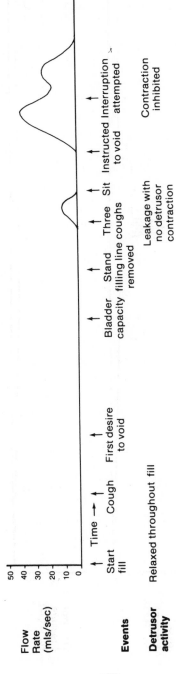

Figure 3.11(b) *Genuine stress incontinence.*

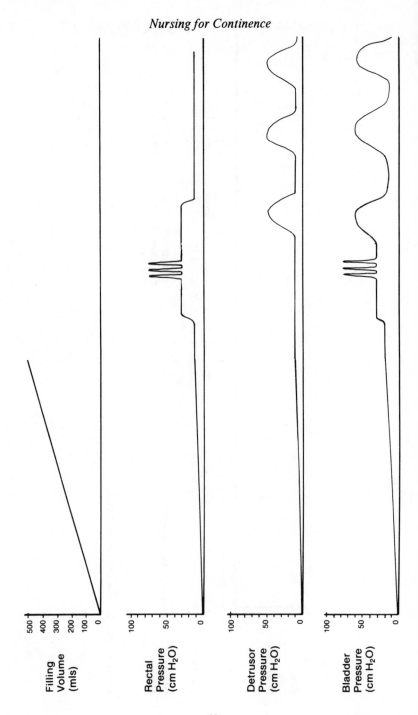

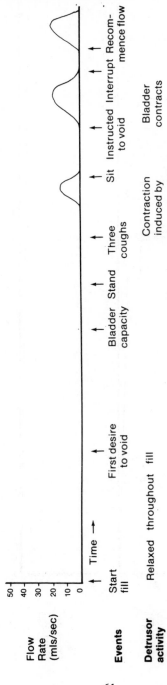

Figure 3.11(c) *Detrusor instability induced by stress.*

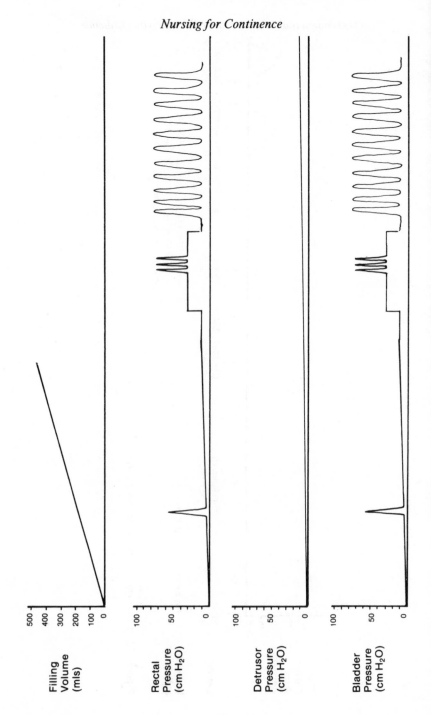

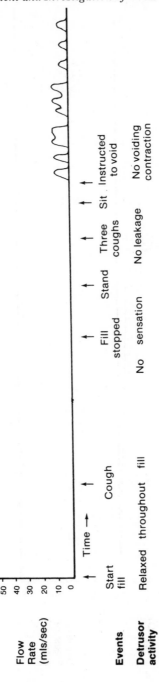

Figure 3.11(d) *Atonic bladder.*

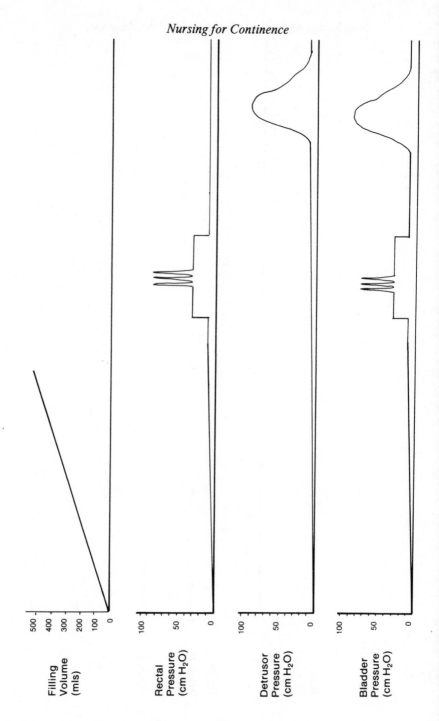

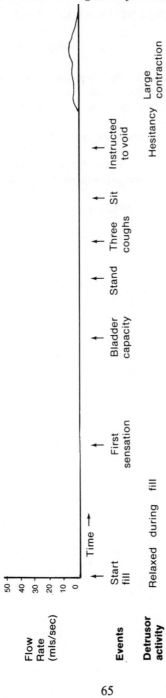

Figure 3.11(e) *Outflow obstruction.*

REFERENCES AND FURTHER READING

Clay, E. C., 1978. 'Incontinence of urine'. *Nursing Mirror*, 146, 10, 36–38, 146, 11, 23–24.

Griffiths, D. J., 1980. *Urodynamics: the Mechanisms and Hydrodynamics of the Lower Urinary Tract.* Adam Hilger, Bristol.

Incontinence Action Group, 1983. *Action on Incontinence.* Kings Fund Centre, London.

Mandelstam, D. (ed.), 1980. *Incontinence and its Management.* Croom Helm, Beckenham.

Norton, C. S., 1980. 'Assessing incontinence'. *Nursing*, 1, 18, 789–791.

Norton, C. S., 1984. 'The promotion of continence'. *Nursing Times Supplement*, 80, 14, 4–10.

Stanton, S. L. (ed.), 1978. 'Gynaecological urology'. *Clinics in Obstetrics and Gynaecology*, April, 5:1.

Stanton, S. L. (ed.), 1984. *Clinical Gynaecologic Urology.* Part 2, 'Investigation'. C. V. Mosby Company, St. Louis.

Chapter 4

Treating and Managing Incontinence

The principles involved in treating or managing urinary incontinence which are relevant to any incontinent person are given in broad outline in this chapter. Later chapters cover aspects relevant to specific groups, so the present chapter should be considered in conjunction with as many of the later chapters as apply to any individual patient.

All interventions must be planned in the light of information gathered during the assessment and investigation of the individual's incontinence, as outlined in Chapter 3. The aim of treatment is to alter those factors which have been found to be causing incontinence. Management is aimed at ameliorating the effects of being incontinent upon the individual and his carers. Obviously treatment, aimed at 'cure', and management, aimed at improved coping, cannot be completely separated, and usually both will be implemented at the same time.

Sometimes one single intervention is indicated. This tends to be the case for the younger, otherwise fit, incontinent person where the sole cause is a bladder dysfunction. In other cases a complex inter-related package of interventions, involving several different team members, will be needed. There are very few people for whom any attempt at cure is inappropriate – usually only the critically or terminally ill and the profoundly demented. For the majority, cure or considerable improvement is possible and should be attempted. However, it is certainly likely in the foreseeable future that there will be a substantial minority who cannot regain total continence. For these people efficient and appropriate management methods are essential, if incontinence is not to be a handicap in its own right.

NURSING MANAGEMENT AND ADVICE

The nurse has a key role in giving advice and support to the incontinent individual and his family or carers, whether the problem is

67

being treated or has been found to be intractable. Minimising the effect of incontinence upon the patient and his surroundings means that most can lead a relatively normal life despite their incontinence. Wherever the nurse is advising the patient or relatives about the condition, the basic principles of teaching should always be remembered. Information should only be imparted in small amounts, and repeated often, if it is to be retained. Written back-up is useful, as this can be read later. (See Feneley and Blannin, 1984, and Mandelstam, 1977, for useful patient books.)

EXPLAINING THE PROBLEM

Many people are very ignorant about how their body functions, and their understanding of incontinence is based on misconceptions. A clear explanation of the working of the lower urinary tract and why it has gone wrong will help the patient to participate in therapy. The patient who understands his condition can be much more active in tackling his problems, yet the tendency of many nurses and doctors is still to remove that responsibility from the individual by not imparting sufficient information. Where the patient himself is incapable of learning, the rest of the family can usually benefit from teaching. (See Norton, 1983, for a review of the nurse's role in patient teaching for continence.)

Information will also help the patient and his family to come to a decision about treatment options, where alternatives exist. For instance, if surgery is suggested the patient has the right to know what is involved, what the chances of success are, and what risks or side-effects there may be. Although the surgeon would discuss these, it is often the nurse to whom the patient turns for detailed information. Many people are reluctant to ask what they feel might be 'obvious' questions or to reveal their fears or ignorance, and the nurse must allow time and offer appropriate prompts to help the patient to make an informed decision. It must be up to the individual to decide how far he wishes to pursue treatment.

PSYCHOLOGICAL SUPPORT

The nurse's attitude and approach towards the incontinent patient should demonstrate that she does not see incontinence as a stigma to be ashamed of, but as a symptom to be dealt with. The guilt, shame and embarrassment felt by many incontinent people (and their relatives on their behalf) can be eased by a nurse who treats her patient with respect. This is vital, as so many incontinent people lose all self-esteem and confidence and become pessimistic about the possibilities of improvement. The nurse must feel unembarrassed about discussing intimate details if the patient is to be able to express all his fears and worries. The nurse may be tempted to brush away unfounded fears quickly, but a brusque 'Of course you don't smell', or 'Nobody thinks you are a baby', or 'Of course your husband/wife still finds you attractive' will do little to reassure. It may also cause the nurse to fail to understand the real problem – what constitutes a problem to the patient may not be obvious to the nurse. Unless a close and trusting relationship is developed, the nurse may never be able to empathise with her patient and realise what help he needs.

Support may take different forms. Sometimes just listening is enough. A sounding-board for the expression of feelings, especially frustration and anger, can be useful in defusing tensions within a family. Often, the individual can be helped to reach his own solutions by a nurse who listens, encourages, and prompts full expression of the problems, rather than by a nurse who talks continuously and leaves no space for any response.

Improving the incontinent person's self-image is an essential element in enabling him to cope with incontinence. If inter-personal or sexual relationships have suffered because of the incontinence, considerable encouragement is often needed before the patient will attempt to resume normal relationships. Fear of rejection is powerful and restricting. Relatives who are caring for a heavily incontinent person at home are in as much need of support as the patient. It is not difficult to see how the relatives might come to feel inadequate and hopeless, guilty that they are not doing all they could, especially if comparing themselves with a nurse who appears very competent and able to cope. The district nurse visiting under such circumstances may usefully spend as much time reassuring and listening to the carer as giving nursing care to the patient.

Some incontinent people are in need of more formal psychological help, and where the nurse does not have the appropriate training or expertise it may be better to consider referral to a counsellor, psychiatrist, psychologist or sexual dysfunction clinic, rather than attempt support alone. The nurse must recognise her own limitations and the point at which another professional would be of greater help to her patient.

SKIN CARE

Good skin care is essential for anyone who is incontinent. Regular incontinence can be associated with dermatitis, and in conjunction with a factor such as friction, with the development of pressure sores in vulnerable individuals. Both urine and faeces can cause direct skin irritation. They also provide a damp and warm environment which is ideal for the proliferation of potentially pathogenic micro-organisms. However, it must be said that the majority of incontinent people do not have sore perineal skin for most of the time, and only a minority develop significant soreness, infection or pressure sores. Even the doubly incontinent immobile person does not inevitably suffer skin problems. Skin health depends to a large extent on general health, especially upon a balanced diet and adequate fluid intake. Those who are very sick or debilitated are much more vulnerable to skin breakdown. The nurse can offer much useful advice on diet and general health care to help prevent or treat skin problems.

The most important element of skin care is thorough cleansing of the entire genital area (and any other skin in contact with urine or faeces) at least twice a day. Ideally a bath or shower should be taken daily. This is not always practicable and a good wash must sometimes suffice. Warm water and a mild soap should be used. Heavily scented soaps may provoke a skin reaction and may cause discomfort if the skin is already sore. After washing, the skin must be gently but thoroughly dried with a soft towel. Healthy skin should not require any creams or lotions. If the skin is known to be vulnerable, a simple barrier cream such as zinc and castor oil may be used. Any cream should be used sparingly – too much may make the skin surface soggy and actually increase the risk of problems. Skin should be patch-tested before using a proprietary cleansing or barrier product, as so many people are sensitive to one or more of the many different substances contained in these products. If unsure whether soreness is because of incontinence or the cream supposedly used to protect the skin, one should apply the product to a separate area of skin (for example, on the back) and observe for skin reaction over several hours. Where the skin is already sore, a cream with combined barrier, analgesic, and healing properties (e.g. Sudocrem) is often found to promote healing. Talcum powder is best avoided as it can irritate, especially if strongly perfumed, and tends to form lumps when dampened by urine or sweat, causing encrustations in the groin skin folds.

If the skin is becoming sore, factors other than the incontinence should not be forgotten. An aid or pad may be the cause. A pad may have a rough surface, or an appliance be too tight-fitting. Plastic in contact with wet skin is an especial source of trouble, and plastic pants should be avoided. Some patients' skin may be sensitive to the materials of a pad or appliance, and inflammation may be caused by an allergic reaction. Pressure or friction is often more significant than urine. In elderly women a sore vulva may be the result of atrophic vaginitis rather than incontinence.

If the skin has become very sore and the surface has broken down, sometimes the only viable method of healing it is by using an indwelling catheter to control the incontinence. This should never be used solely for nursing convenience (see Chapter 15), but may be unavoidable for severe skin problems.

CONTROLLING ODOUR AND SOILING

Odour is one of the greatest fears of incontinent people (Norton, 1982). Sufferers may restrict their activities and social contacts, not because of obvious leakage, but because they worry about smelling. In Western society natural odours have become taboo, and vast amounts of money are spent on disguising everyday smells in the home and on the body. If perspiration is considered unacceptable, how much more is this true of excreta? Modern man (or woman) does not like to be reminded of bodily necessities. People who smell of urine or faeces are considered socially unacceptable, and are avoided. Most people assume that those who smell must neglect themselves and be unclean in their habits.

For most incontinent people their worry is unfounded, as they do not smell. This does not prevent them from worrying that they do, and repeated reassurance is often needed. Freshly voided urine has only a faint odour, provided that it is not too concentrated and is not infected. If adequate attention is paid to personal hygiene even regularly incontinent people should not smell. Only if urine is allowed to linger does odour become offensive, because of breakdown of urine constituents on contact with air. Where possible, soiled pads and clothing should be changed soon after incontinence has occurred. Appliances present less of a problem, as urine is contained in a bag. Washing the skin is not usually necessary or feasible after each episode of incontinence but it must be done regularly (see Skin Care, above). Faecal incontinence represents a more difficult problem (see Ch. 14).

If urine is particularly offensive the patient should be encouraged to increase fluid intake, and the urine must be tested for infection. One of the most effective methods of preventing odour is to ensure that the incontinence is well contained by a good pad or appliance, and that clothing and the environment are protected from contamination. When a pad is removed it should be put immediately into a sealed container such as a plastic disposal bag with tie seal, or a bin with a well-fitting lid. Appliances should be washed thoroughly each day. Soiled clothes, beds, chairs or carpets are often the source of a lingering smell. Some materials (notably wool) seem to exacerbate the problem. Furniture can be difficult to clean effectively if soiled. Often this is overcome by using a plastic mattress or cushion cover, and linoleum rather than carpet. However, this can make the bed or chair uncomfortable and many people do not wish to live in an environment where everything is plastic-covered. This is true both in the person's own home and in an institutional setting. It may be difficult to strike a balance between adequate protection and an acceptable environment. Probably the best answer is to minimise the risk of contamination by using the best available aids (see Chapter 13). Odour can become very offensive if clothes or furniture are not noticed to have been soiled and thus are not cleaned. Slippers are often a particular source of smell – well-fitting shoes which can be wiped easily are usually preferable to soft carpet-slippers, which are difficult to clean properly.

Not all incontinent people are able to maintain high standards of hygiene, especially those who both live alone at home and are disabled. Even a good wash may be impossible for many people without help. In a proportion of District Health Authorities help with bathing can only be given weekly, or even fortnightly. This is obviously insufficient to prevent odour. Some people have great problems in washing soiled clothes and bedding. Home help or laundry services may be able to help (see Chapter 11), but people often just dry soiled items without first washing them. The nurse can advise that this is not a good idea, but without adequate social services there may be no other solution. The problem may be eased by advising the patient to buy clothes or bedding made of materials which are easy to launder and quick to dry. (Dark clothing also tends to show wet patches less and so reduces embarrassment.)

Some people have very poor standards of personal hygiene and seem unconcerned about odour or cleanliness. The nurse may be in the difficult position of receiving complaints from those around the patient, while the individual is oblivious of any problem. Sometimes the nurse has either to discuss this frankly with the patient, or risk his being banned from activities or ceasing to have visitors. Incontinent people may be sacked from work, stopped from going to a luncheon club, or no longer invited to visit relatives because of a smell that they themselves appear to be unaware of.

In some instances odour comes to dominate the incontinent person's environment – whether his own home or an institution. Sometimes the only answer is to cleanse everything completely, often discarding carpets and mattresses, and start again. In severe cases the Public Health Department may be called in to fumigate the home. The tell-tale odour that used to be associated with geriatric wards is becoming less common, but may still be encountered, especially where high-quality aids are not used. The main focus of the nurse's attention should be control of the incontinence rather than the smell it causes.

Several proprietary deodorants are available for use where smell is a problem (see Chapter 11).

FLUID INTAKE

Fluid balance is often disturbed in incontinent people. Most adults drink between one and two litres of fluid per twenty-four hours, but this may be considerably increased with exercise, heat, or sociable drinking. It is necessary to produce a minimum of 500ml of urine in twenty-four hours to permit adequate excretion of waste products.

Many incontinent people restrict their fluid intake in an attempt to control incontinence. If taken to extremes this can lead to dehydration and even to electrolyte imbalance and confusion, especially in the elderly. Others suffer almost continuous thirst, which can become most unpleasant. Fluid restriction should usually be discouraged and the individual instructed to drink as he feels the need or desire.

It is possible that fluid restriction may actually be counter-productive, for several reasons. A very low urine production, if combined with frequent voiding, will mean that the bladder is never expanded to its full capacity. While this is unlikely to reduce bladder capacity physically, it is likely to lower bladder sensitivity to a smaller habitual volume. In those prone to cystitis, a urinary tract which is only irregularly and infrequently emptied and flushed out may encourage re-infection. Low fluid intake will worsen any tendency to constipation. It is also possible that very concentrated urine may actually irritate the delicate mucosa of the bladder trigone and aggravate feelings of urgency and frequency.

Incontinent people should be encouraged to consume a reasonable fluid intake (1–2 litres per day). However, the times at which this is taken are unimportant, so timing can be manipulated accordingly. If the patient is most troubled by incontinence while out in the daytime, it may be wise for him to drink the bulk of the intake after returning home. If nocturia and nocturnal enuresis are the main problem, some fluid restriction may be advisable in the evening. However, this does not justify the extremes that some people (including nurses) practise – for example no fluids after afternoon tea for those with nocturnal enuresis. This is both inhumane and frequently ineffective. All too often it becomes a 'ward policy' and is continued unthinkingly, even if it has never been proved effective, and even if the patient still wets every night.

Certain fluids may create special problems for some individuals. Some people find that either tea or coffee has a rapid diuretic effect for them and is better avoided. Others say white wine is fine but red wine is not. It is usually a matter of trial and error to discover these idiosyncracies.

Patients with an indwelling catheter are usually encouraged to drink extra fluids (2–3 litres per day – see Chapter 15). However, some other people may also seem to be drinking excessively. This often follows advice, from medical or lay sources, on avoiding cystitis. At times people are discovered habitually drinking more than five litres per day. This will obviously make incontinence more of a problem, and very few people actually need this large amount.

INCONTINENCE AIDS

The nurse will usually be the person to advise the incontinent person on the appropriate use of aids to control incontinence. This subject is covered in Chapter 13.

BOWEL MANAGEMENT

Poor bowel function may affect bladder control and is often the major problem in faecal incontinence. The nurse must help the individual to establish a programme to regulate a good bowel habit and teach him and his family how to maintain this. Chapter 14 gives suggestions on bowel management.

THE ENVIRONMENT AND PHYSICAL ABILITIES

An environment geared to the individual's needs, especially if he is physically disabled, will often enable incontinence to be avoided. Chapter 9 includes suggestions as to how the environment might be modified to improve continence, and ways in which the individual's physical abilities may be maximised to help him cope with bladder function.

THE ROLE OF THE DOCTOR

The role of the nurse and doctor can overlap to a considerable extent in helping the incontinent patient. Much of the advice described above, and bladder training (pages 80–92), might equally well be initiated by a nurse or doctor. Some specific medical and surgical treatments, aimed at remedying the underlying bladder dysfunction, may also be used.

DRUG THERAPY

Many different drugs have been prescribed to help people with urinary incontinence. Often the results have been disappointing, and there is certainly no 'wonder drug' for any type of incontinence. However, there are some which may be useful for carefully selected and accurately diagnosed patients.

Detrusor instability
The control of unstable bladder contractions and urge incontinence, by using a drug either to relax the detrusor muscle or inhibit reflex contractions, seems to offer one of the most promising areas. Table 4.1 (overleaf) lists the drugs most commonly used. As can be seen, if the drug is given in large enough doses to be effective, most of them have side-effects which can be so troublesome as to make the treatment unacceptable.

In trials, placebo effect has been found to be considerable. It seems likely that the general advice, concern, and bladder training which usually goes with the prescription of these medications may be as important as the drug itself.

This is not to say that these drugs are not very useful, especially in the initial stages of treating a patient with urge incontinence or nocturnal enuresis. Their effect can help with the introduction and acceptance of a bladder-training programme. For some people the

Table 4.1: Drug Therapy for the Unstable Bladder

Drug name	Usual dose	Method of action	Common side-effects	Comments
Imipramine (Tofranil)	10–25mg nocte initially Up to 25–50mg t.d.s.	Anticholinergic (blocks reflex contractions) + alpha agonist (increased urethral resistance) + ? Central effect	Dry mouth Constipation Drowsiness Postural hypotension (possible falls in the elderly)	Tricyclic antidepressant. Use with great care in glaucoma and *never* with monoamine oxidase inhibitors.
Propantheline (Pro-Banthine)	15mg t.d.s.	Anticholinergic	Dry mouth Blurred vision Constipation	More usually used for gastro-intestinal disorders, e.g. peptic ulcer.
Emepronium bromide (Cetiprin)	200mg t.d.s. or 400mg nocte	Anticholinergic	Dry mouth Blurred vision Constipation	Poorly absorbed if taken orally. Tendency to cause ulceration of mouth and oesophagus.
Flavoxate hydrochloride (Urispas)	200mg t.d.s.	Smooth muscle relaxant	Nausea Dry mouth Blurred vision	
Oxybutinin (Ditropan)	5mg t.d.s.	Anticholinergic	Very dry mouth Constipation	Not yet available on prescription in UK.

drug alone will be effective in curing the incontinence, although there is a tendency for relapse if medication is withdrawn. Used in combination with a retraining programme, the patient can often be weaned from the tablet once a normal bladder pattern has been attained. Imipramine is probably the most acceptable first choice for therapy, combining reasonable success rates with minimal side-effects if used in low doses.

Because the purpose of all these drugs is to reduce bladder contractions, they should be used with great care with patients who have a voiding difficulty, since urinary retention may be precipitated. Careful prior assessment will have included a measurement of residual urine; drug therapy should be introduced with great caution in cases where the volume is over 100ml.

Genuine stress incontinence

Some drugs have been used in an attempt to prevent stress incontinence by increasing urethral tone. Phenylpropanolamine (Eskornade) and ephedrine are the most commonly used, especially in children, and are thought to act on the alpha receptors in the urethra.

Oestrogen replacement therapy can improve urethral resistance in the atrophic urethra (see Chapter 8).

Outflow obstruction

Drug therapy may be used to relieve outflow obstruction. Phenoxy-benzamine is the most commonly used but may have very troublesome side-effects (tachycardia and postural hypotension), and must be used with great caution.

Atonic bladder

Where the bladder will not contract sufficiently to ensure complete bladder emptying, drug therapy may be tried to improve the force of the voiding contraction. Carbachol, bethanechol and distigmine bromide have all been used, with limited success. All may produce unacceptable side-effects if used in effective doses.

Other drugs

Other drugs may be useful in treating factors influencing bladder function, for instance appropriate antibiotics to treat a urinary tract infection or laxatives to treat or prevent constipation.

Many drugs may exacerbate a tendency to incontinence, and the physician should be aware that drugs prescribed for many conditions may be adversely affecting bladder function (see Table 2.2). A policy of choosing medication with minimal effects on continence should be pursued, where possible, with all people vulnerable to incontinence. For example, a slow-acting diuretic, in a divided dose, may allow those with urgency to avoid urge incontinence. An analgesic may be preferable to night sedation for those who wet the bed at night and need pain relief.

SURGERY

Urinary incontinence is unfortunately sometimes the result of surgery, usually urological or gynaecological, but also major pelvic or spinal operations. This iatrogenic incontinence may be caused by neurological or mechanical damage to the bladder-control mechanism, leading to any of the bladder dysfunctions.

As with drug therapy, surgery designed to *remedy* incontinence is best considered according to the bladder problem it aims to solve. (For details of surgical techniques see Stanton and Tanagho, 1980.)

Detrusor instability
None of the several surgical approaches which have been tried to treat the unstable bladder has gained widespread use. In experienced hands surgery can be effective, but the condition tends to recur and it is difficult to envisage general acceptance. Cystodistension (stretching the bladder under general anaesthetic), bladder transection and selective sacral neurectomy are all presumed to act by disturbing the neurological pathways which control uninhibited contractions.

Genuine stress incontinence
Where stress incontinence is caused by an incompetent sphincter mechanism in women, the experienced gynaecologist can offer either vaginal or suprapubic surgery with a very high expectation of success (see Chapter 6). In men a damaged sphincter may be repaired by a prosthesis (see Chapter 7). These are the most commonly performed operations in the treatment of incontinence and, if diagnosis and surgical technique are correct, excellent results are usual.

Outflow obstruction
Surgery may be used to relieve outflow obstruction, for example, to remove an enlarged prostate gland (see Chapter 7), divide a stricture or widen a narrow urethra (urethrotomy). If any of these are done by an inexperienced surgeon there is a risk of rendering the patient incontinent.

Severe intractable incontinence

Some people with severe intractable incontinence which has failed to improve, despite all treatment efforts, may wish to consider major surgery to correct this. For those with a damaged urethra a neo-urethra can be constructed from a bladder flap, or else an artificial sphincter can be inserted (see Chapter 7). In some instances a urinary diversion into an ileal conduit with a stoma can bring tremendous benefits, especially in women. Although a seemingly drastic solution, a stoma is often much easier to cope with than an incontinent urethra, because an effective appliance will contain the urine. Extensive pre-operative counselling is essential for people considering this option, and wherever possible an experienced stoma care nurse should become involved with the patient and family.

THE CONTRIBUTION OF OTHER TEAM MEMBERS

In a well-integrated multidisciplinary team, each member has a role to play in helping incontinent people. Although the strict differentiation of roles is artificial, each has his own sphere of expertise which may be of use to a particular patient.

The physiotherapist, whether in hospital or community, can assess the patient's mobility and dexterity, and implement a treatment plan if these could be usefully improved. Extending the range and strength of movements may make it easier for the patient to get to, or on to, the lavatory. A demonstration of safe lifting techniques may prevent accidents or strains in cases where a relative is involved in aiding transfers. Where a walking-aid or wheelchair is used the physiotherapist can ensure that these are optimal for the individual's needs. For stress incontinence a patient may be referred for pelvic-floor exercises (with or without faradism or interferential therapy, see Chapter 6).

The occupational therapist is skilled in helping the individual towards independence in the activities of daily living, including personal hygiene and toileting. Techniques may be used to improve function, or aids provided to maximise the abilities present. Modifications to clothing, alternatives to the lavatory, and implements to aid washing or dressing can all be tailored to the specific needs of the individual.

Social workers are ideal people to mobilise and co-ordinate resources in the community, because of their extensive knowledge of local facilities. It may be possible to arrange modifications to the home, attendance at a day centre or luncheon club, home-help or laundry services, voluntary services and financial assistance, according to the individual's needs (see Chapter 11).

A psychologist is of particular help with patients of impaired mental abilities (handicapped or demented), and where incontinence is felt to be a behavioural problem. A detailed psychological assessment will enable a treatment plan to be made to meet the needs of the individual. The psychologist may also be involved in treating psychologically disturbed patients and in counselling patients, families, and other staff members. In the community the community psychiatric nurse may fulfil this role.

A great variety of other professionals may become involved with the incontinent person when appropriate. The chiropodist can make a great difference to mobility. The optician may help to improve the patient's vision and make mobility safe. The dietitian or dentist may be involved in ensuring that the patient can eat a healthy diet.

The nurse must be aware of the potential contribution of all of these professionals and know when referral is appropriate. Often restoration of continence is only one aspect of a comprehensive rehabilitation programme designed to achieve maximum possible independence for each patient.

BLADDER TRAINING

'Bladder training' or 'retraining' is a much misused and misunderstood term in nursing. Nearly every nurse who has incontinent patients under her care will, if asked, claim to be practising 'bladder training'.

It is very common to read in nursing care plans: 'Problem – incontinence; planned action – bladder training'. There is rarely any elaboration on what is meant by the term, how such training is to be carried out, or what the ultimate goal may be (other than a very general 'the patient will regain continence'). Bladder training has come to be seen as a panacea for incontinence, a treatment which is universally applicable. Often in practice the 'training' amounts to nothing more than reminding the patient or taking him to the lavatory every two hours.

Bladder training is indeed a useful nursing tool, but only when used appropriately by a nurse who understands the technique. Several different types of toileting programmes may be distinguished and used in different circumstances. The most important element for success is that the correct regime is selected for each individual patient and situation. Success is highly unlikely if every incontinent person is treated identically. A thorough prior assessment will identify those patients who should benefit from bladder training and which method is most appropriate. It is important that any other factors contributing to the incontinence have already been diagnosed and are being treated – for instance, a urinary tract infection or constipation – as these will certainly impair the success of a programme.

Bladder training is most suitable for people with the symptoms of frequency, urgency, and urge incontinence (with or without an underlying unstable bladder), and for those with a non-specific incontinence which they are unable to account for and which seems to 'just happen'. Elderly patients in institutional care very often have this non-specific incontinence. This chapter outlines bladder training for the mentally alert. Programmes for the elderly, mentally infirm, and the mentally handicapped are covered in Chapters 8 and 12 respectively.

Patients with a bladder dysfunction other than an unstable bladder are unlikely to benefit from bladder training. A woman with an incompetent urethral sphincter, and consequent stress incontinence, will not be able to regain continence by manipulating her lavatory visits. She may, by excessive frequency, be able to keep the bladder relatively empty so that only a little urine is in it, but her underlying problem will remain. Even if she has just passed urine the next time she coughs she is likely to leak. Similarly, the person with urinary retention and overflow incontinence will seldom be helped by training. This emphasises the importance of thorough assessment and accurate diagnosis prior to the implementation of any treatment programme.

BLADDER RETRAINING FOR URGE INCONTINENCE

The aim of bladder retraining is to restore the patient with frequency, urgency and urge incontinence to a more normal and convenient micturition pattern. Ultimately voiding should occur only every three to four hours (or even longer), without any urgency or incontinence. When the bladder is known or thought to be unstable, drug therapy is often combined with the bladder training.

The key to success is accurate record-keeping and frequent professional contact and support. Retraining may be used with success with inpatients or outpatients. Occasionally patients may be admitted to hospital specifically to undergo a retraining programme (gynaecologists in particular may use inpatient programmes: e.g. Frewen, 1978; Jarvis and Millar, 1980).

The patient must fully understand and enthusiastically participate in this treatment. There is no doubt that it can be very difficult for the patient to follow. A lot of time must be spent at the outset explaining the programme in detail, emphasising that only the patient himself can make it a success. Initially, a clear description of normal bladder function and why and how it has gone wrong should be given. If, for whatever reason, the patient cannot or will not co-operate, there is little point in attempting this type of bladder retraining.

It must be explained that the bladder for some reason (usually unknown or because of some neurological disease) has become 'over-active' and 'over-sensitive'. The individual may have experienced urge incontinence. The natural reaction to this embarrassing experience is to try to prevent it happening again. Usually the patient will develop a habit of rushing to the lavatory at the first hint of bladder filling, in order to pre-empt an accident. Since the bladder fills continuously (and most people can sense some urine in the bladder if they think about it) it is not difficult to see how a vicious circle of passing urine more and more frequently can develop. The person anxious about incontinence is likely to interpret any slight bladder sensation as an urgent need to pass urine, immediately interrupting his activities to seek a lavatory. Anxiety or worry merely enhances the sensation of urgency. In extreme cases, someone's life may become completely ruled by the need to pass urine every ten to fifteen minutes. Few people get to this unhappy state, but many visit the lavatory every hour or half-hour throughout the day. In spite of this level of frequency, they may also experience urge incontinence – especially if they have an unstable bladder. If someone gets up and rushes to the lavatory while the bladder is contracting he is very likely to be incontinent – women are more vulnerable than men because of a lower urethral resistance. 'Key-in-the-lock' incontinence may develop – the person can hang on while rushing urgently home, but wets on the front doorstep while fumbling to get the door unlocked, or gets to the lavatory but is incontinent while trying to remove clothing.

Bladder training aims to restore the individual's confidence in the bladder's ability to hold urine, and to re-establish a more normal pattern. Initially the patient should keep a baseline chart for three to seven days, recording how often he passes urine and when incontinence occurs. This is then reviewed with the nurse or doctor supervising the programme, and an individual regime is devised. The purpose is gradually to extend the time interval between toilet visits, encouraging the patient to practise hanging on, rather than to give in to the urgency. Initially the times chosen should not be too difficult to achieve. The times may be at set intervals throughout the day (e.g. every hour or two hours), or variable, according to the individual's pattern as shown by the baseline chart. For example, someone taking diuretics in the morning might need to go hourly in the morning, every hour-and-a-half in the middle of the day, and two-hourly in the evening. Someone who has fixed time commitments (e.g. working, or taking children to school) might need times to fit in with travelling or meal breaks. Every attempt should be made to make the programme as convenient as possible – it is much more likely to be followed. If the baseline chart reveals a definite pattern to the incontinence it may be possible to set toileting times to anticipate this. If someone is always wet at 3.30 p.m., a good time would be 3 p.m.

The patient is therefore set a pattern of toileting times throughout the day. Usually no times are set at night, even if nocturia or nocturnal enuresis are problematic. The patient is instructed to pass urine as necessary at night. Sometimes it is useful to set an alarm clock to anticipate a known peak wetting time. This is often unnecessary, because nocturnal problems often resolve themselves once daytime frequency has returned to normal.

The patient is instructed to pass urine at the set times and to attempt to hang on in between. Sometimes the provision of a suitable pad or appliance will add to confidence and mean that if incontinence does occur, the results will not be too disastrous. If urgency is experienced the patient must sit or stand still and try to suppress it, rather than rush immediately to find a lavatory. A normal fluid intake is encouraged, as the aim is to have the patient continent and able to drink whatever he wants.

As the patient achieves the target intervals, without having to go prematurely or leaking, the intervals should gradually be lengthened. The speed of progress in this is very individual and will depend on many variables, such as initial severity of symptoms, motivation, and the amount of professional support. Outpatients will often need to remain at one time interval for one to two weeks before this is extended at the next clinic visit. Inpatients may have their programmes reviewed much more often, even daily in some cases. It is usual to increase the time interval by fifteen minutes to half-an-hour at a time, but again this will vary considerably and some people will manage leaps of an hour at a time. Any times which seem particularly difficult should be adjusted to suit individual needs – e.g. someone who habitually drinks four mugs of tea at breakfast will probably never achieve a four-hourly voiding interval in the morning. The intelligent outpatient who understands fully the purpose of the programme will often adjust his own time intervals and be able to progress considerably between clinic visits.

Once the target of three- to four-hourly voiding without urgency has been achieved, it is useful to carry on keeping the charts and set times for at least another month to prevent relapse. Some people take several months to achieve this, whereas others may need only a few weeks. There seems to be no way of predicting how long bladder training is likely to take for each individual. Figure 4.1 shows a series of charts monitoring the progress of a woman with an unstable bladder. Filling in the charts consistently is vital in assessing progress, and gives the patient useful feedback that results are positive.

An alternative to bladder training by pre-set time intervals is to instruct the patient gradually to extend the time interval between the first sensation of urgency and actually passing urine. Instead of setting a pattern to aim for, the patient tries to hang on for ever-increasing intervals after feeling the need to go, and so gradually spaces out his toilet visits. For example, someone with severe urgency might be asked to count to ten slowly before starting for the toilet. Once this was achieved without incontinence, the count should be raised to twenty, then thirty, then sixty. If urgency is less severe, the patient might start by waiting ten minutes, then twenty minutes, then half-an-hour. The highly motivated patient will often see for himself how the ticks on the chart are gradually spacing out, and set his own target to aim for.

Some people find that practising pelvic-floor exercises (see Chapter 6) helps to suppress urgency. It is important not to underestimate how difficult it is to ignore the sensation of urgency if you know that you might wet yourself. Many patients will be tempted to give up the bladder training or refuse to push themselves. Often bladder training will contradict other advice they have been given – for example, many children are taught that it is bad to hold on for too long. However, it is one of the few hopes that people with urge incontinence have of regaining continence, and every attempt must be made to encourage and support their efforts.

More use could be made of mutual support between patients, in the form of groups, than is currently practised.

Treating and Managing Incontinence

Continence Chart

Week commencing _____ Name **Mrs Bell**

Please tick in LEFT column each time urine is passed
Please tick in RIGHT column each time you are wet

	Monday		Tuesday		Wednesday		Thursday		Friday		Saturday		Sunday	
6 am	✓				✓					✓	✓	✓✓	✓	
7 am	✓	✓	✓	✓	✓	✓	✓		✓	✓	✓		✓	
8 am			✓		✓				✓✓					✓
9 am	✓		✓				✓	✓			✓		✓	
10 am		✓	✓✓		✓				✓	✓	✓		✓	
11 am	✓				✓		✓					✓		
12 pm	✓✓		✓	✓	✓	✓	✓		✓		✓		✓	
1 pm			✓		✓✓		✓						✓✓	✓✓
2 pm	✓				✓				✓		✓✓		✓✓	✓
3 pm	✓	✓✓	✓				✓			✓	✓		✓	✓
4 pm		✓		✓	✓		✓		✓				✓	
5 pm	✓		✓✓								✓	✓		
6 pm							✓		✓				✓	
7 pm	✓		✓		✓	✓			✓		✓			
8 pm			✓						✓					
9 pm	✓						✓		✓		✓		✓	
10 pm			✓		✓				✓					
11 pm							✓		✓					
12 am	✓		✓		✓		✓				✓		✓	
1 am											✓			
2 am	✓	✓												
3 am														
4 am													✓	✓
5 am														
Totals	13	6	14	3	13	3	10	2	12	5	13	4	14	6

Special Instructions

Baseline charting. Please record your pattern of visits to the lavatory and wetting, without intentionally changing them this week.

Figure 4.1 *Series of charts showing progress of a patient on a bladder-training programme. (a) Baseline week. The patient is asked to record micturition and incontinence.*

85

Continence Chart

Week commencing **Week 1**   Name **Mrs Bell**

Please tick in LEFT column each time urine is passed

Please tick in RIGHT column each time you are wet

Time	Monday		Tuesday		Wednesday		Thursday		Friday		Saturday		Sunday	
6 am			✓											
(7 am)	✓		✓		✓		✓		✓					
(8 am)	✓		✓		✓	✓	✓		✓		✓		✓	
9 am	✓				✓									✓
(10 am)	✓		✓				✓	✓	✓		✓		✓	
(11)	✓		✓		✓		✓				✓		✓	✓
12 pm	✓	✓			✓	✓			✓	✓				
(1 pm)	✓		✓	✓	✓		✓		✓		✓		✓	
(2)	✓		✓		✓		✓		✓		✓		✓	
3 pm													✓	✓✓
(4 pm)	✓		✓		✓		✓		✓		✓			
5 pm													✓	
(6 pm)	✓		✓		✓		✓		✓✓	✓	✓			
7 pm														
(8 pm)	✓	✓	✓		✓		✓		✓		✓		✓	
9 pm														
(10 pm)	✓		✓				✓		✓		✓		✓	✓
11 pm					✓								✓	
(12 am)	✓		✓		✓		✓		✓					
1 am											✓			
2 am														
3 am														
4 am							✓							
5 am														
Totals	12	3	11	2	12	2	12	1	12	2	10	0	11	4

Special Instructions

Pass urine only at the times indicated at left. Try to hang on in between. If you have to make additional trips to the lavatory, record these also.

Figure 4.1(b) *The nurse and patient review the baseline chart and work out a pattern of visits to the lavatory (times circled in left-hand column).*

Continence Chart

Week commencing __Week 2__ Name __Mrs Bell__

Please tick in LEFT column each time urine is passed
Please tick in RIGHT column each time you are wet

	Monday	Tuesday	Wednesday	Thursday	Friday	Saturday	Sunday
6 am		✓					
(7 am)	✓	✓	✓	✓	✓	✓	
8 am					✓✓ ✓		
(9 am)	✓	✓	✓	✓			✓
10 am			✓		✓	✓ ✓	
(11 am)	✓	✓	✓	✓	✓	✓	✓
12 pm							✓
(1 pm)	✓	✓	✓	✓	✓	✓	✓
2 pm	✓ ✓✓						
(3 pm)	✓	✓	✓	✓	✓	✓	✓
4 pm					✓		✓
5 pm		✓	✓ ✓✓			✓ ✓	
(6 pm)	✓	✓	✓	✓	✓ ✓	✓	✓
7 pm							
8 pm	✓						✓✓ ✓
(9 pm)	✓	✓	✓	✓	✓	✓	✓
10 pm							
11 pm			✓ ✓		✓		✓
(12 am)	✓	✓	✓	✓	✓	✓	
1 am	·						
2 am							
3 am				✓			
4 am						✓	
5 am							
Totals	10 2	10 0	11 3	9 0	12 2	10 2	10 1

Special Instructions

Pass urine only at the times indicated at left. Try to hang on in between.

Figure 4.1(c) *At the weekly review the patient agrees to try to slightly extend the time gap between visits to the lavatory.*

Continence Chart

Week commencing ___Week 4___ Name ___Mrs Bell___

Please tick in LEFT column each time urine is passed
Please tick in RIGHT column each time you are wet

	Monday		Tuesday		Wednesday		Thursday		Friday		Saturday		Sunday	
6 am														
(7 am)	✓		✓		✓		✓		✓		✓			
8 am														
(9 am)	✓		✓		✓	✓	✓		✓		✓		✓	
10 am					✓	✓								
(11 am)	✓		✓	✓	✓		✓				✓		✓	
12 pm									✓	✓				
(1 pm)	✓		✓		✓		✓		✓		✓		✓	
2 pm														
(3 pm)	✓		✓		✓		✓		✓		✓		✓	
4 pm														
5 pm									✓					
(6 pm)	✓		✓		✓		✓		✓		✓		✓	
7 pm										✓				
8 pm													✓	
(9 pm)	✓		✓		✓		✓		✓		✓			
10 pm														
11 pm							✓							
(12 am)	✓		✓		✓		✓		✓		✓		✓	
1 am														
2 am														
3 am														
4 am														
5 am														
Totals	8	0	8	1	9	2	9	0	9	2	8	0	7	0

Special Instructions

Pass urine only at the times indicated at left. Try to hang on in between.

Figure 4.1(d) *By the fourth week the patient is usually managing to 'hang on' until the set time, and incontinent episodes have become rare.*

Continence Chart

Week commencing **Week 5** Name **Mrs Bell**

Please tick in LEFT column each time urine is passed
Please tick in RIGHT column each time you are wet

	Monday		Tuesday		Wednesday		Thursday		Friday		Saturday		Sunday	
6 am									✓	✓				
(7 am)	✓		✓		✓		✓		✓		✓			
8 am													✓	
9 am	✓								✓					
(10 am)	✓		✓		✓		✓		✓		✓		✓	
11 am														
12 pm			✓											
(1 pm)	✓		✓		✓		✓		✓		✓	✓	✓	
2 pm											✓	✓		
3 pm		✓												
(4 pm)	✓	✓	✓		✓		✓		✓		✓		✓	
5 pm														
6 pm														
7 pm	✓			✓			✓	✓						
(8 pm)	✓		✓	✓	✓		✓		✓		✓		✓	
9 pm														
10 pm														
11 pm		✓		✓							✓			
(12 am)	✓		✓		✓		✓		✓				✓	
1 am														
2 am														
3 am														
4 am														
5 am														
Totals	8	3	7	3	6	0	7	2	8	1	7	2	6	0

Special Instructions

Pass urine only at the times indicated at left. Try to hang on in between.

Figure 4.1(e) *Extending the time interval still further to achieve a 'normal' micturition pattern causes a slight relapse of incontinence . . .*

Continence Chart

Week commencing **Week 8** Name **Mrs Bell**

Please tick in LEFT column each time urine is passed

Please tick in RIGHT column each time you are wet

	Monday		Tuesday		Wednesday		Thursday		Friday		Saturday		Sunday	
6 am					✓									
7 am	✓		✓				✓		✓					
8 am											✓		✓	
9 am					✓									
10 am	✓													
11 am			✓				✓		✓		✓			
12 pm														
1 pm													✓	
2 pm	✓		✓		✓		✓							
3 pm									✓					
4 pm											✓		✓	
5 pm	✓		✓											
6 pm							✓							
7 pm			✓						✓					
8 pm			✓								✓		✓	
9 pm	✓						✓							
10 pm									✓		✓			
11 pm	✓				✓								✓	
12 am			✓				✓		✓		✓			
1 am														
2 am														
3 am														
4 am														
5 am														
Totals	6	0	6	0	5	0	6	0	6	0	6	0	5	0

Special Instructions

Maintain a gap of at least three hours between visits to the toilet.

Figure 4.1(f) . . . *which has disappeared again by the 8th week. By now the patient need not stick rigidly to set times, merely ensuring that she always waits at least three hours between lavatory visits.*

SET INTERVAL TOILETING

Much of what goes under the name of 'bladder training' in fact does nothing to train the bladder, and consists solely of reminding or taking a patient to pass urine at set intervals. This is most commonly practised in residential homes and long-stay hospitals. The intervals chosen may be time-related (e.g. every two or four hours) or else be related to events (e.g. before or after taking meals, drinks, or drugs). Often such programmes are applied indiscriminately to all residents, or at least to all those who are incontinent. As everyone's bladder functions differently, such a programme will at best catch some incontinence before it occurs. Usually it is completely unrelated to individual needs. Hopefully, with the advent of more individualised patient care, such a rigid regime for a whole group will be recognised as both ineffective and time-consuming.

However, set patterns are useful for selected patients. Those with a very poor memory, who tend to simply forget about their bladder until it is too late, may benefit from fixed time interval reminders or a standing instruction always to visit the lavatory after meals. Sometimes an alarm clock or a set interval timer (e.g. Contilarm-Pearson) may serve as a reminder if there is no one around. Patients with impaired bladder sensation may also need to be instructed to pass urine by the clock, rather than waiting for sensation, if they are to avoid overflow incontinence. Patients with advanced dementia, for whom all attempts at continence have failed, may be kept dryer by set interval toileting (see Chapter 8).

HABIT RETRAINING

Habit retraining has been described as a method of training the elderly in hospital (Clay, 1978). A baseline chart is kept to determine the individual's pattern of continence and incontinence (as with bladder training). A programme of toilet times is then worked out to anticipate incontinence. Toileting times are therefore worked out for each individual in a ward, rather than treating everyone the same. Once continence is achieved, the time intervals may then be lengthened. In practice such a programme is much more likely to keep patients continent than set-interval toileting for all, and may retrain some bladders. Possibly the biggest benefit, certainly to long-stay patients, is to 'retrain' the staff to recognise individual toileting needs, rather than taking everyone at the same time. (See Chapter 11 for toileting regimes in residential and hospital care.)

BIOFEEDBACK

Biofeedback is a sophisticated form of bladder training for patients with detrusor instability. The patient must be reasonably intelligent and motivated, and the treatment is only available in urodynamic clinics. By connecting the patient to the urodynamic equipment, as for a cystometrogram (as described in Chapter 3), filling the bladder slowly and showing the patient what is happening to bladder pressure, many patients are helped in learning to inhibit their unwanted bladder contractions (Cardozo et al., 1978). Usually six to ten one-hour sessions are needed with a skilled therapist, so the treatment is expensive and time-consuming. Further research is warranted to bring this technique to greater numbers of people.

REFERENCES AND FURTHER READING

Cardozo, L., Stanton, S. L., Hafner, J., Allen, V., 1978. 'Biofeedback in the treatment of detrusor instability'. *British Journal of Urology*, 50, 250–254.

Clay, E. C., 1978. 'Incontinence of urine'. *Nursing Mirror*, 146, 10, 36–38; 146, 11, 23–24.

Feneley, R. C. L., Blannin, J. P., 1984. *Incontinence: Patient Handbook*. Churchill Livingstone, Edinburgh and London.

Frewen, W. K., 1978. 'An objective assessment of the unstable bladder of psychosomatic origin'. *British Journal of Urology*, 50, 246–249.

Jarvis, G. J., Millar, D. R., 1980. 'Controlled trial of bladder drill for detrusor instability'. *British Medical Journal*, 281, 1322–1323.

Mandelstam, D., 1977. *Incontinence*. William Heinemann Medical Books, London.

Norton, C. S., 1982. 'The effects of urinary incontinence in women'. *International Rehabilitation Medicine*, 4, 1, 9–14.

Norton, C. S., 1983. 'Training for urinary continence'. In: Wilson-Barnett, J. (ed.), *Patient Teaching*. Churchill Livingstone, Edinburgh and London.

Stanton, S. L., Tanagho, E. A., 1980. *Surgery of Female Incontinence*. Springer-Verlag, Berlin.

(See also General Reading (Appendix 3) for reviews of treatments.)

Chapter 5

Incontinence in Childhood

The achievement of continence is an important developmental milestone. Society places responsibility for this achievement upon a child's parents. The mother who has failed to 'potty-train' her infant by the expected age will often feel either that she has somehow failed in her maternal duties or that her child is backward or retarded. Child-rearing practices vary over time and fashions tend to go in cycles, alternating between starting training as early as possible and using virtually no training at all.

The incontinent child is often the recipient of hostility and may feel rejected. Once past that crucial age at which continence is expected, it is no longer acceptable to crouch in a gutter or pass urine against a wall in public view. What was once viewed as 'quaint' behaviour becomes 'incontinence' as the toddler approaches school age. He comes to realise that it is considered shameful to lack bladder control. Parents may react with anger in an attempt to disguise their own guilt and embarrassment. If the child really has no control, punishment cannot be avoided and he may become shy, anxious and withdrawn.

At school the incontinent child often suffers ridicule and humiliation at the hands of classmates. During the course of his own toilet training the continent child will often have adopted attitudes that wetting is infantile and naughty. Having provided proof that he has acquired grown-up habits and left behind such baby-like behaviour, he may mercilessly tease his less fortunate peers. Other parents may be very lacking in understanding and tolerance, instructing their own child not to play with the 'smelly' or 'dirty' incontinent child. Many seem by their attitude to blame the parents for negligence in not bringing the child up properly or not bothering enough to toilet-train him. Most teachers and schools are more enlightened, but some make life difficult for the incontinent child. Strict routines that only allow toilet visits during official breaks may make a child with limited ability to hang on actually incontinent. Such a situation will certainly increase anxiety.

Some nursery schools will not take children until they are reliably continent. Sometimes a handicapped child is obliged to attend a special school, not because his intellectual ability or emotional needs are different, or because of his handicap, but because of his incontinence.

TOILET TRAINING

It is likely that 'training' does more to teach the child socially acceptable toileting behaviour, and to recognise the permitted places, than to train the bladder itself. The complex neuromuscular control necessary for continence and voluntary micturition cannot be taught by a parent. Natural maturation, especially of the central nervous system, is the most important factor in acquiring control. It is likely that even with no training at all children can eventually control micturition (although not necessarily using the 'correct' receptacle). One consequence of neuromuscular immaturity is that continence at birth is impossible. Mothers who start potty-training at three months may 'catch' some urine in the pot, but fail to realise that this is purely by chance and that the baby cannot yet do this reliably. Up to 80% of parents are attempting some sort of toilet training by the infant's first birthday. This is far too early for most infants, and it is hardly surprising that so much anxiety is aroused over what must inevitably become a prolonged battle.

The optimum time to attempt training is probably around the second birthday, depending on the child's general developmental achievements. Ideally he should be able to walk and follow simple instructions, and have some speech and basic feeding skills. At this point the training is most likely to be easy and rapid, although the prospect of dispensing with nappies and gaining social approval for early achievement are powerful temptations to start much sooner.

Most children are toilet trained without professional intervention. However, many nurses are asked for advice, either officially as a health visitor, district or clinic nurse, or socially as a relative or friend. The best advice is to wait until the child is ready and then to train fairly intensively, choosing if possible a time when little else is going on (e.g. avoiding Christmas, or family holidays). This is preferable to random and premature attempts over a long period. The child should be taken out of nappies and put into dry pants so that he learns to appreciate the difference between wet and dry. Clothing and underwear should be easy for the child to remove independently. Frequent prompts and potting are combined with immediate reward (physical or verbal) for passing urine, and disapproval or rebuke for accidents. Excessive punishment is counter-productive, because it raises anxiety, thereby decreasing the learning potential. Mild reprimands do no harm provided that the child has the potential ability to avoid them in future. The child should be given clear and repeated explanations of what is required. It may be useful to temporarily increase fluid intake in order to increase the number of learning opportunities.

Some very intensive toilet-training methods have been devised, for example 'in less than a day' (Azrin and Foxx, 1974). These are difficult to operate without experienced professional supervision.

If a planned attempt conducted at an appropriate time fails, it is best to stop trying, put the child back into nappies, and try again after an interval of two to three months, by which time he may be ready. A parent or sibling can sometimes help the child to learn by demonstrating appropriate toilet behaviour.

Adults take continence so much for granted that it is easy to forget how many different skills are involved. It is not simply a matter of passing urine while sitting on the potty. The child must learn to consciously perceive the need to micturate, and be able to monitor the state of the bladder both asleep and awake. Once the need is appreciated, micturition must be postponed until an appropriate receptacle is reached. It is not always easy to know what an acceptable place is, especially if the surroundings are unfamiliar. For example, boys must learn to recognise a urinal as appropriate, as well as a lavatory, but a bidet as inappropriate. Girls must learn only to pass urine behind a closed, preferably locked, door, except in the countryside when they can go behind a bush. Boys can go in front of other boys, but not in front of girls, and must defaecate in private. The pre-literate child is naturally unable to read signs on public conveniences. The child must also learn to open doors, remove clothing, use lavatory paper, flush the toilet, and wash his hands. Once in position the stream must be started voluntarily. Not until all these skills have been mastered can the child be independent at toileting. The final skill in the sequence is not gained until the child is about five years old, when the ability to pass urine in the absence of any sensation of needing to do so is perfected. This is most important socially as it enables anticipatory micturition: being able to empty the bladder 'just in case', e.g. prior to a class or a journey. This is vital to prevent inconvenient interruptions to activities and makes everyday life much more orderly.

If professional help is sought for failure to become dry it is usually best, after an initial assessment to exclude serious pathology, simply to reassure the parents that there is unlikely to be anything wrong and that the child is not stupid or naughty; the parents should be advised to give up and try again in a few months. Explanation of a simple reward system (e.g. a cuddle immediately upon performance) can be helpful. If repeated attempts have failed, it is useful to keep a chart to monitor progress and put the problem into perspective (Figure 3.2). Sometimes established points of conflict can be changed, for instance by buying a new pot or by using a different room, or having a different person to do the training. Confidence and optimism, with emphasis on positive achievements rather than failures, will usually resolve most problems.

PERSISTENT DIURNAL INCONTINENCE

Daytime wetting sometimes persists until school age. It is less common than bedwetting (see below), and the two often go together. If the child is continuously dribbling this should be fully investigated, as there may be a voiding difficulty which could threaten renal function. Wetting more usually takes the form either of urge or stress incontinence. Many children wet on the odd occasion when they have been so engrossed in playing that they repeatedly ignore warnings from the bladder. This can be safely dismissed as being of no pathological significance.

Most children would grow out of daytime wetting eventually, without any formal intervention. However, because incontinence can be such a nuisance and embarrassment, both to child and parents, it is usually worth trying to hasten continence, provided that both the child and the parents want help and are eager to co-operate.

If the problem is frequency, urgency and urge incontinence, treatment is very similar to adult bladder training (see Chapter 4). A time should be chosen when full attention can be devoted to the training programme (e.g. during a school holiday). The training can either be strictly by the clock, or by delaying micturition once sensation is felt. In the former method the child is reminded to pass urine once every half-hour on the first day, and this interval is increased by half-an-hour per day until voiding is $2\frac{1}{2}$–3-hourly. In the latter method, after he first feels the need to go on the first day, he must count to ten before setting out for the lavatory. On day 2 he counts to twenty, on day 3 he must wait half a minute. This should be gradually increased until ten minutes elapse between the onset of sensation and going to pass urine. With both these methods some accidents should be expected and tolerated. A chart should be kept throughout the training period to monitor progress and to give both child and parents feedback on success. A parent, or other trainer, must be enthusiastic and willing to devote about a week to the programme, giving maximum encouragement and optimism to the child throughout. It is vital that any programme is consistently carried out by all concerned. Frequent small rewards can be offered during the training period. The promise of one big reward for success should be avoided. It can put a considerable stress upon the child to know that he will not get a new bicycle if he fails, and this may be counter-productive. Fluids should not be restricted during the training period. Usually the child is well motivated by the desire to be rid of the problem.

A different but complementary approach to controlling urgency is to practise when actually at the lavatory. This is useful for the child who tends to wet at the last moment. The child should get into position ready for micturition and then count to ten before allowing the stream to start. Once he can do this he should count to ten at the door as well. Once this is mastered he should count ten before starting out for the lavatory, at the door, and once in position. This is aimed at increasing confidence in the ability to control the bladder. Nothing exacerbates urgency so much as the fear that it will lead to wetting.

Sometimes a pants alarm (Figure 5.1, Nottingham Medical Aids) is useful in bladder training, especially if the child is unaware when incontinence is occurring. These alarms have the dual function of interrupting the stream, as the child is startled when the buzzer sounds, and also of alerting him to the fact that he is wet. The small sensor is worn inside the pants in a mini-pad, or between two pairs of pants. This is obviously unsuitable for use anywhere but at home.

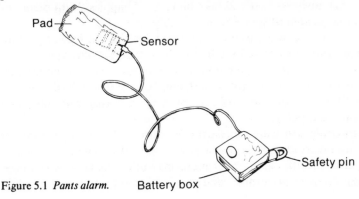

Figure 5.1 *Pants alarm.*

Occasionally persistent urgency and frequency may be caused by a urinary tract infection, especially in girls. If the child has dysuria, smelly urine, or fails to respond to bladder training, it is always worth getting a urine specimen checked for infection.

Although training should always be started with great optimism, the child should not be blamed or punished if it should fail. Instead he needs reassurance that he will manage it soon, and can try again next holiday.

Stress incontinence – that is, leakage upon physical exertion – is usually caused by a weakness of the pelvic-floor component of the urethral sphincter. The treatment of choice is pelvic-floor exercises, described in detail in Chapter 6. The child should be taught to interrupt the urine midstream at every micturition and then to practise pelvic-floor contractions regularly throughout the day. A few girls seem to be born with a congenitally weak or open bladder neck. For a few this resolves spontaneously at puberty, but corrective surgery is sometimes required if incontinence is troublesome.

Some girls suffer 'giggle incontinence', whereby they start to leak when they laugh but may continue to leak until the bladder is completely empty. This is probably a combination of stress incontinence and an unstable bladder, and can be treated by combining a bladder-training programme with pelvic-floor exercises.

NOCTURNAL ENURESIS (BEDWETTING)

Most children become dry at night between the third and fourth birthday. Dryness is usually established over a fairly short period. Once the child has had a few dry nights the parent should explain that dryness is now expected and take him out of nappies. With plenty of encouragement most soon become reliably dry.

However, one in ten five-year-olds still wet the bed regularly. With no treatment this gradually falls to 5% of ten-year-olds and 1%–2% of adults. It is twice as common in boys as girls, has strong familial tendencies, and is associated with stressful events in the third to fourth year of life. In girls a urinary tract infection is occasionally the cause (Kolvin et al., 1973).

Bedwetting can cause considerable distress. The sheer volume of washing involved is great, especially if more than one child wets or if washing facilities are poor. Parents may think the child is just lazy, or even doing it on purpose, and in a few instances this leads to child abuse. When the child is older he is often prevented from staying overnight with friends for fear of it happening, and school or family holidays become difficult. If the bedwetting persists into adolescence and adult life, it may make the individual reluctant to leave home or form lasting relationships. Occasionally the problem is not mentioned, even to a prospective marriage partner, and the enuretic may break off the engagement rather than face the embarrassment of telling his or her partner. In fact, luckily, enuresis often spontaneously stops upon change of circumstances, such as starting to share a double bed. Many sufferers will not take the risk.

Lifelong enuresis has been implicated as a factor on the road to homelessness (Stone, 1973). Attitudes of partners, flatmates, landladies and hostel wardens may lead to repeated rejections and descent into vagrancy. It is not difficult to imagine how unpleasant it must be to share a bed with someone who is enuretic, and why it is a major deterrent to forming lasting relationships.

Treatment for nocturnal enuresis is usually delayed until it has become enough of a problem for both the parents and the child to want some action to be taken. Seldom should it be considered before the age of five. Sometimes very simple remedies are effective. A clear explanation of bladder function should be given. Popular myths, such as deep sleep, laziness or intentional wetting should be dispelled. It is quite common for a child only to wet at home, not when sleeping elsewhere (e.g. at the grandparents' house), and parents may interpret this as the child being able to control it if he wanted to. Every attempt should be made to put the problem into perspective if the situation has become tense and wetting is a point of conflict. For instance, most children do not realise that there is likely to be at least one other enuretic in their class at school, so that they are not alone, or a freak. Many do not know that they have an excellent chance of growing out of it and are very unlikely to continue bedwetting for much longer.

Sometimes an obvious mistake can be identified, such as failing to pass urine before retiring to bed. If the child also has daytime frequency and urgency, the training programmes outlined above are useful in increasing functional bladder capacity. Some parents practise 'lifting' – they awaken the child to empty his bladder on their way to bed. This may prevent wetting, and probably does no harm, although it does little to train the child. Occasionally it can be counter-productive as the child comes to expect it and never develops the ability to hold urine all night. He may even become conditioned to wet at the sound of footsteps coming up the stairs, or, if lifting is at a regular time, this may become the time at which he wets when not lifted. If lifting is used it is wise to vary the time and who does it, so that it does not become a trigger for wetting.

Star charts (Figure 5.2) can be a very useful aid. The child is encouraged to keep his own chart. A common system is to get one star (say, a blue one) for each dry night. For three consecutive dry nights a gold star may be stuck on. Emphasis should be on positive achievement and no 'black marks' should be used for wet nights. Care should be taken to explain to the parents that if a child does respond to a star chart this does not mean that he simply was not trying hard enough before. Response to a simple reward does not imply that the same result could have been obtained by effort alone.

Anticholinergic medication is sometimes used in conjunction with a star chart. Imipramine (Tofranil) is the most common. This often results in very rapid cure, but unfortunately relapse is usual when medication is withdrawn. The incidence of accidental poisoning with imipramine is reportedly very high, with children easily mistaking the bright tablets for sweets, and this provides a very strong contra-indication to its use. It may also cause or aggravate a tendency to constipation.

ENURESIS ALARMS

If bedwetting is problematic and does not respond to simple measures the treatment of choice is the enuresis alarm or 'bed buzzer'. This is an extremely effective method if well supervised, and will cure 80% of bedwetters. Unfortunately in practice it is all too often improperly used and poorly supervised. Many school nurses, paediatric departments, health clinics and health visitors have a stock of buzzers to lend out, but many will simply give it to the family with little explanation of how or why it should work, with an instruction to 'come back in three months'. Understandably few children are cured and treatment is often abandoned long before it could become effective.

The amount of disruption and extra work occasioned by the use of a buzzer should not be underestimated. It is essential that parents and child are well motivated for success. If there is any suspicion of child abuse the treatment should be particularly closely supervised and supported.

The use of the alarm must be explained to the child in language appropriate to his level of understanding. It is usual to describe it as helping him to learn bladder control. Most alarms consist of two mesh

Name _____

Date commenced _____

Remember: Always go to the toilet before going to bed. In the morning stick on a blue star for a dry night. For the third dry night in a row stick on a GOLD star.

	1st Week	2nd Week	3rd Week
Monday	☆	☆	☆
Tuesday	☆	☆	☆
Wednesday	☆	☆	☆
Thursday	☆	☆	☆
Friday	☆	☆	☆
Saturday	☆	☆	☆
Sunday	☆	☆	☆
	4th Week	5th Week	6th Week
Monday	☆	☆	☆
Tuesday	☆	☆	☆
Wednesday	☆	☆	☆
Thursday	☆	☆	☆
Friday	☆	☆	☆
Saturday	☆	☆	☆
Sunday	☆	☆	☆

Figure 5.2 *Star chart.*

mats with connecting leads to a battery box. The equipment should be set up as in Figure 5.3. A waterproof layer is placed directly on the mattress, followed by the bottom mat, either covered with a sheet or in a pillowcase. On top of this comes the top mat covered with a sheet or drawsheet. It is essential that the two mats are separated by a clean dry layer of material.

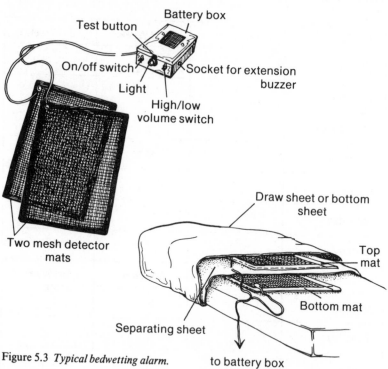

Figure 5.3 *Typical bedwetting alarm.*

Most alarms have a test button so that the equipment can be tested before retiring. The box should be placed far enough away from the bed so that the child cannot reach out to turn the buzzer off and then roll over and go back to sleep again. Ideally he should have to get right up out of bed to switch the alarm off. A normal (not restricted) fluid intake should be allowed and the bladder emptied prior to retiring. If acceptable, no nightclothes should be worn from the waist down – any clothing delays urine from reaching the sensor mats. Where feasible, sleeping in a room alone is ideal so that siblings are not disturbed. If this is not possible, this generally does not matter too much and an older brother or sister may even assist the child.

When the child wets, urine passes through the sheets and an electrical circuit is completed between the two mats. This causes the buzzer to sound. The usual response is to interrupt micturition and to wake up. The child often has difficulty in waking, especially during the first week. Sometimes the alarm can cause panic or fright at first, and where possible the parents should sleep within earshot. If the child does not wake they should go to him and wake him while the buzzer is still sounding. It is most important that he should wake to the sound of the alarm. Once awake the child should get up and attempt to finish off passing urine in the toilet. Younger children will almost certainly need help to re-make the bed and re-set the alarm. Older children may manage alone, especially with the aid of a night-light. Re-setting is important in case of a second wet. In the morning a chart should be filled in to record the size of the wet patch and whether there was any urine left to pass in the lavatory (Figure 5.4, overleaf).

Most children need fifteen to twenty wet nights before they learn either to wake up before the bladder empties (and so get up to pass urine) or alternatively to hold urine all night. Either of these is a sign of success. Progress is usually indicated by the wet patch getting smaller and more urine being left in the bladder to finish off.

There are some common problems which can lead to the failure of therapy. The equipment itself may be faulty, especially if heavily in use on loan. Each user will need new batteries and usually new mats. Sometimes the connector leads can become loose or the batteries flat during treatment. False alarms can occur if the mats become frayed or touch. If the child fails repeatedly to wake to the sound of the buzzer, models are available with louder signals, or the box can be put in a biscuit tin to amplify the sound. The child can be conditioned to wake to the alarm by using it to wake him in the morning. He may also be taught to interrupt micturition to the sound of the buzzer if it is sounded when he is passing urine by day – the automatic reaction is to jump and stop. Sweating may cause false alarms. An extra layer of material between the mats, or less bedding or a cooler bedroom, may remedy this. Nylon sheets should be avoided.

It is not clear why the enuresis alarm is effective. Some workers have claimed that it is classical conditioning – the child learns to pair the sensation of a full bladder with the conditioned response of waking and voiding. Others have suggested it may be avoidance learning – the child learns to avoid the unpleasant event of being woken by the buzzer. It is difficult to prove or disprove either theory.

Vibrating alarms which can be placed under the pillows or against

Name .... **Week Commencing** ....

Please fill in this chart each morning

	Was the bed wet? (Yes or No)	Did the child wake to pass urine in the night? (Yes or No)	Fill in this section if alarm sounded in the night			
			At what time(s) did the alarm sound?	Did the alarm wake the child? (Yes or No)	Size of wet patch S = small, M = medium, L = large	Did the child have more urine to pass in the toilet? Write no, small, or large amount
Monday						
Tuesday						
Wednesday						
Thursday						
Friday						
Saturday						
Sunday						

Figure 5.4 *Detailed treatment record chart.*

the collar-bone are available for deaf children or for those who sleep in a dormitory or with siblings. Some alarms employ only a single mat which makes the equipment much simpler to set up, although with some models this makes the mats less robust and causes more false alarms. The pants alarm already shown in Figure 5.1 can also be used at night inside a pad, and again is discreet and easy to set up. Boys might object to wearing a pad and may prefer to wear the sensor between two pairs of pants.

A bed buzzer can be used both with mentally and physically handicapped children. Obviously more parental supervision is required. Care must be taken with the mentally handicapped that the buzzer is not seen as pleasurable, so that wetting is intentional to trigger the alarm. It sometimes happens that a child will sit on the bed in the daytime and wet on purpose to create the buzz.

Treatment with the alarm usually takes three to four months. During this time it is wise to keep a regular check on the family to iron out any problems as soon as they arise and to keep up motivation. A home visit to see the equipment actually set up is useful if problems occur. Once the bed has been reliably dry for four weeks the use of the alarm can be discontinued.

Roughly one-third of children will relapse at some time after conclusion of successful treatment. This relapse rate can be lowered considerably (to about 12%) by using 'overlearning' (Morgan, 1978). This means that once the child has been dry for fourteen consecutive nights he should deliberately drink one to two pints of extra fluid before going to bed. This will often result in wetting recurring for a few nights, but the child usually soon becomes dry again and now has a 'margin of error'. Once there have been two dry weeks on the high fluid intake the extra fluid and the alarm are discontinued. If wetting does not start to diminish after two weeks of overlearning it should be abandoned and the child put back to a normal fluid intake, with the alarm, until he becomes dry again.

If relapse occurs this does not mean the buzzer will not work a second time, and it should be used again. The child who has relapsed once does in fact have the same chance as first-timers of becoming dry and not relapsing again.

The enuresis alarm has been extensively used and researched with childhood bedwetters (Kolvin et al., 1973; Morgan, 1978). Its use with adult enuretics is little documented. It is certainly well worth trying with life-long bedwetters. Whether it has any role to play with the elderly who develop secondary enuresis remains to be seen.

CONGENITAL ABNORMALITIES

Certain congenital abnormalities of the urinary tract may be the underlying cause of incontinence in childhood. Minor abnormalities may well be overlooked unless a careful physical examination is carried out on a child presenting with continuous or very frequent wetting day and night. Occasionally, congenital deformities are not picked up in childhood and persist undiagnosed into adult life.

Epispadias and hypospadias (Figure 5.5)
Epispadias is a condition where the urethra opens on the upper surface of the penis. It can vary from an abnormally wide meatus to a complete split of the penis. It is rare in females, where the clitoris and pubic bone are split. Treatment is surgical repair, but only one-half of boys achieve complete continence.

Hypospadias, an opening of the urethra on the undersurface of the penis, is much commoner, affecting 1 in 600 boys. The boy tends to

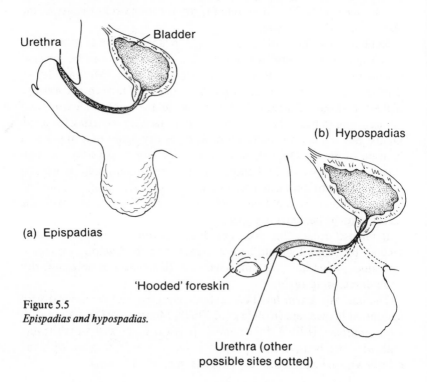

Urethra

Bladder

(b) Hypospadias

(a) Epispadias

'Hooded' foreskin

Figure 5.5
Epispadias and hypospadias.

Urethra (other possible sites dotted)

have a 'hooded' foreskin, no normal erections, and a urinary stream which is passed backwards, between the legs. Again, treatment is surgical and usually gives good results in both continence and sexual function.

Ectopic ureter

The ureter, instead of inserting into the bladder at the trigone, may enter the urethra directly. If this is below sphincteric level a continuous dribbling incontinence will result. Sometimes this is associated with duplication of the upper urinary tract, with one ureter in the correct place and the second being ectopic. In this case the child will be able to pass urine normally but also suffer dribbling.

Urethral valves

Some boys are born with urethral valves which prevent proper bladder emptying, leading to retention with overflow incontinence. Usually diagnosed early in life, the baby often presents in renal failure with a poor urinary stream and a urinary tract infection. This is a serious condition and must be corrected surgically. Occasionally, boys who have had such surgery develop continence problems at a later date.

Ectopia of the bladder

This is a rare and obvious condition where the abdominal wall fails to develop over the bladder, which consequently opens directly onto the skin at birth. The bladder has to be surgically reconstructed or the ureters diverted into an ileal conduit.

Parents of children with congenital abnormalities usually need a great deal of support. They often feel guilty for somehow having caused the deformity. They are usually very worried that the child will never be 'normal'. They may fear for later sexual identity and function. Careful explanations and realistic reassurance are vital. Some repairs are done in several stages, involving the child in repeated hospital admissions at a vulnerable stage. The child or his siblings may suffer emotionally, whether or not the parents stay in hospital with the child. If the condition is not urgent, repair is often left until he can cope better psychologically (e.g. after school age). However, this may result in several years of both incontinence and feeling abnormal. Although long-term physical results are often excellent, the nurse has an important contribution in ensuring that the patient adjusts psychologically to the fullest possible extent.

REFERENCES AND FURTHER READING

Azrin, N. H., Foxx, R. M., 1974. *Toilet Training in Less than a Day.* Pan Books, London.

Hutchings, J., Williams, B., 1978. 'Toilet training: 1. The normal child'. *Journal of Community Nursing*, 2, 3, 22–23.

Kolvin, I., Mac Keith, R. C., Meadows, S. R. (eds.), 1973. *Bladder Control and Enuresis.* William Heinemann Medical Books, London.

Lovibond, S. H., 1964. *Conditioning and Enuresis.* Pergamon, Oxford.

Meadow, R., 1980. *Patient Handbook: Help for Bed-wetting.* Churchill Livingstone, Edinburgh and London.

Morgan, R. T. T., 1978. 'Relapse and therapeutic response in the conditioning treatment of enuresis: a review of recent findings on intermittent reinforcement, overlearning and stimulus intensity'. *Behavioural Research and Therapy*, 16, 273–279.

Morgan, R. T. T., 1981. *Childhood Incontinence.* William Heinemann Medical Books, London.

Smith, P. S., 1980. 'Questions mothers ask about toilet training'. *Nursing*, 1, 18, 800–801.

Stone, H., 1973. *Adult Bedwetters and Their Problems.* Cyrenians, Canterbury.

Chapter 6

Female Incontinence

While both men and women may suffer incontinence for all the reasons outlined in Chapter 2, there are a few conditions specific to the female which are described in greater depth in this chapter. Stress incontinence is particularly common amongst women; all nurses have an important role in teaching preventive measures and in teaching, counselling and giving care to sufferers. It will often be a nurse who teaches and supervises a programme of pelvic-floor exercises, or the use of occlusive devices. For women who opt for surgery, pre-operative counselling and post-operative care and support are a major contribution to successful outcome. The midwife and health visitor will encounter many women with incontinence problems in pregnancy and immediately after childbirth.

GENUINE STRESS INCONTINENCE

There is considerable confusion in terminology over the use of the phrase 'stress incontinence'. In fact it can be used to describe a symptom or as a medical diagnosis. When describing a symptom it denotes the experience of leaking urine upon physical exertion (physical, *not* emotional, 'stress'). As a diagnosis it refers to incontinence caused by incompetence of the urethral sphincter – a failure of the urethra to maintain continence when stressed by raised intra-abdominal pressure.

The symptom and diagnosis do not always coincide in one person. Leakage upon effort could be caused by an unstable bladder; for example, a cough might trigger a bladder contraction, thus mimicking an incompetent sphincter. Likewise people in retention can experience overflow incontinence upon effort. Conversely, a patient whose underlying bladder problem is an incompetent sphincter may complain of symptoms more suggestive of bladder instability, including frequency and urge incontinence. It is for this reason that a history can be

109

most misleading in diagnosing the cause of incontinence, and in many cases urodynamic investigation will be required (see Chapter 3).

In the remainder of this chapter the term 'stress incontinence' is used to refer only to incontinence caused by a weak or incompetent sphincter. In the International Continence Society's definitions this is referred to as 'genuine stress incontinence'.

MECHANISM OF STRESS INCONTINENCE

It is thought that stress incontinence in women is caused by an altered anatomical relationship between the bladder and urethra and their muscular supports, notably the pelvic floor.

Figure 6.1 shows the normal relationship. The bladder and proximal urethra sit well supported above the pelvic floor. The intravesical (bladder) pressure is below maximum urethral pressure at rest – a pressure gradient maintains continence. As the bladder is situated inside the abdominal cavity, any rise in intra-abdominal pressure (e.g. on coughing) raises intravesical pressure accordingly, thus tending to squeeze urine out of the bladder. However, because the upper (proximal) urethra is well supported it is also inside the abdominal cavity and therefore subject to the same rise in pressure, tending to squeeze it shut. The pressure gradient is maintained (Figure 6.2). As long as urethral pressure is above bladder pressure at some point along the length of the urethra, continence is maintained.

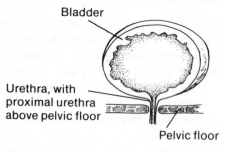

Bladder

Urethra, with proximal urethra above pelvic floor

Pelvic floor

Figure 6.1 *Normal anatomical relationship of bladder, urethra, and pelvic floor: at rest.*

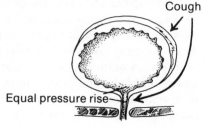

Cough

Equal pressure rise

Figure 6.2 *Normal anatomical relationship of bladder, urethra, and pelvic floor: during a cough.*

Figure 6.3 shows the relationship of bladder and urethra to the pelvic floor in a woman with stress incontinence. The bladder has prolapsed down through the pelvic floor. At rest this woman will be continent, because urethral pressure is above bladder pressure. Bladder pressure is raised when she coughs, but transmission of this pressure rise via the pelvic floor to the urethra is at best partial, at worst nil (Figure 6.4). If the rise in intra-abdominal pressure is high enough, or the urethral pressure low enough for the pressure gradient to be lost, incontinence is the inevitable result.

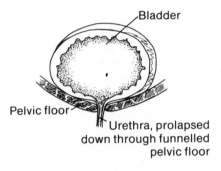

Figure 6.3 *Relationship of bladder, urethra, and pelvic floor in a woman with stress incontinence: at rest.*

Figure 6.4 *Relationship of bladder, urethra, and pelvic floor in a woman with stress incontinence: during a cough.*

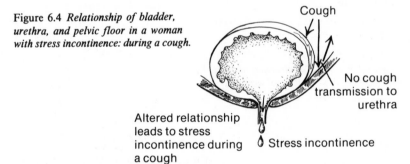

Stress incontinence usually occurs immediately and coincidentally with the onset of effort, and ceases promptly when the activity ceases. It may be mild, only occurring with extreme physical exertion, such as playing squash or trampolining. Or it can be severe, with very minor effort such as walking, talking, or standing up from a chair causing leakage. In pre-menopausal women it tends to be worse in the week before a period, as resting urethral pressure falls with oestrogen withdrawal. Likewise post-menopausal women whose oestrogen level is falling experience an increased tendency to stress incontinence (this is discussed in detail in Chapter 8).

It is possible that the relationship of the urethra to the pubic bone is important to continence. A urethra which is firmly supported up behind the pubic bone is likely to have transmission of intra-abdominal pressure rises augmented by reflection from the bone (Figure 6.5). This theory remains unproven.

The pelvic floor itself contracts reflexly as abdominal pressure is raised (Figure 6.6). This again adds to urethral closure pressure at the crucial time. If, however, the pelvic floor is at an oblique rather than a right-angle to the urethra, the efficiency of this extra margin for continence is impaired (Figure 6.7).

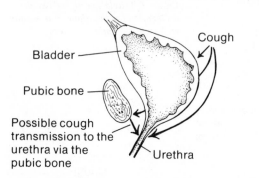

Figure 6.5 *Possible cough transmission to the urethra via the pubic bone.*

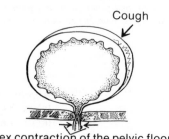

Figure 6.6 *Normal contraction of the pelvic floor with raised abdominal pressure.*

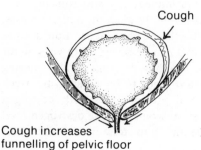

Figure 6.7 *Contraction of the pelvic floor with stress incontinence.*

CAUSES OF STRESS INCONTINENCE

The fact that stress incontinence as described above does not occur in men (who may, however, have sphincter incompetence caused by direct trauma to the sphincter, e.g. post-prostatectomy) highlights the vulnerability of the female anatomy. With such a short urethra and a relatively weak sphincter mechanism, women are very susceptible to stress incontinence. Some surveys suggest that over half of all women experience stress incontinence at some time in their lives. For many it is a regular occurrence which can lead to considerable social restriction: the sufferer becomes unwilling to dance, or even to laugh in public, and comes to dread colds, hay fever, or carrying shopping.

Some females are born with a congenitally weak sphincter mechanism and even an open bladder-neck at rest. This is likely to be the cause of incontinence in girls who wet when they laugh or giggle ('giggle incontinence'). For some this may resolve at puberty, but a few women have never known what it is like to have a good laugh without ending up soaked.

There can be little doubt that childbirth is the most important single factor underlying stress incontinence. Even though nulliparous women do get stress incontinence it becomes much more likely after childbirth, and women who have more than four children have a greatly increased chance of developing it. It is possible that improved obstetric care, especially not allowing a prolonged second stage of labour with consequent prolonged stretching of the pelvic floor, may decrease the prevalence among future generations.

After the menopause many women experience atrophy and sagging of the pelvic supports. It is quite common for stress incontinence to start around the menopause. It is likely that this laxity, added to previous trauma from childbirth, will allow the bladder and urethra to prolapse down through the pelvic floor. The uterus may also prolapse.

Many other factors have been implicated in the causation of stress incontinence, none with totally convincing evidence. Obesity is said to aggravate it, and some women experience improvement in their symptom with weight loss. Repeated heavy lifting may cause trauma to the pelvic floor (although if done correctly this might actually strengthen rather than weaken these muscles). A chronic cough may put repeated stress on the pelvic floor. Habitual straining at stool could cause eventual prolapse. However, the fact that slim, young, childless women experience stress incontinence suggests a basic design fault in the female anatomy.

PREVENTION OF STRESS INCONTINENCE

Studies on the value of preventive health measures are both difficult and expensive to conduct. They have not yet been attempted in relation to the non-fatal condition of stress incontinence, so what follows is conjecture rather than proven fact.

Probably one of the most effective protective measures is conscientious practice of pre- and post-natal exercises. Many women see these exercises as designed to ease delivery and to restore the figure afterwards, as indeed they are. But their value in preventing pelvic-floor laxity is too little emphasised. In the excitement of having a new baby and the exhaustion of sleepless nights, exercise programmes are often deferred or forgotten completely. Many women either do not appreciate, or are not properly taught, the risk to their continence presented by childbirth. Many obstetric units now have a physiotherapist with an additional qualification in obstetrics and gynaecology, who will naturally place great emphasis on pelvic floor re-education post-natally. Where there is no such physiotherapist, the nurse, midwife and health visitor should take on responsibility for teaching, and more importantly, for reinforcing the importance of these exercises, especially in the difficult period after discharge from hospital. Few physiotherapists will be able to see the new mother between discharge and the follow-up appointment, and this is the period when exercises may be abandoned unless the community midwife or health visitor uses her influence to reinforce the teaching started in hospital.

It may well be that greater health awareness will also help to prevent stress incontinence in more general ways. More regular bowel habits, aided by a balanced high-fibre diet, more women taking regular exercise and increased interest in fitness, and an increased demand for hormone replacement therapy in post-menopausal years, may all lead to future generations of women suffering less from stress incontinence. Some keep-fit classes now include pelvic-floor exercises as part of their exercise routine; there is little doubt that an awareness that the pelvic floor exists, and that it can be used and should be protected, should be taught as part of basic health education, ideally beginning at school. Most women are at present totally unaware that such musculature exists.

TREATMENT OF STRESS INCONTINENCE

The ideal time to start treatment for stress incontinence is as soon as the problem arises. Unfortunately many women tolerate it for considerable lengths of time, or until it becomes really troublesome. Public health education could do much to make women realise that they should not expect to leak after having a baby, or as they get older, and that they should seek help for this curable condition. The choice of treatment method will depend upon the severity of symptoms, the degree of concomitant uterine prolapse, and the individual's personal preference.

Pelvic floor exercises
Re-education of the pelvic floor muscles by regular exercise is the best form of therapy for mild to moderate stress incontinence, in the absence of severe uterine prolapse. The patient needs to be well motivated and sufficiently mentally alert to co-operate intelligently and remember to carry out the exercise programme, if it is to be successful. The exercises can be taught by a physiotherapist or a nurse.

There are three groups of muscles comprising the pelvic floor: the levatores ani, the urogenital diaphragm, and the outlet group of muscles. For the purposes of these exercises the levatores ani are the most important. These in themselves have three components: the pubo-coccygeus, the ileo-coccygeus , and the ischio-coccygeus (Figure 6.8. The pubo-coccygeus forms a sling with an anterior gap through which the urethra, vagina and rectum pass. This striated muscle forms the voluntary component of both bladder and bowel control.

Preventive and remedial pelvic floor exercises are essentially identical, although of course once stress incontinence is present they will have to be done more frequently and persistently. Before starting the exercises a careful history should be taken and a thorough explanation of the aims of the exercises given. The following explanation can be adapted to the individual's level of understanding.

It is useful to describe the pelvic floor as a 'hammock' which is suspended between the pubic and tail bones. When this muscle is young and healthy it lies fairly flat and keeps all the body's openings firmly closed. After childbirth (or the menopause, or whatever is appropriate to the patient) the hammock sags and can no longer hold these openings so tightly closed, especially when any additional stress is put upon it. With a cough it just gives way and lets a little urine out. The aim of the exercises is to bring the pelvic-floor muscle back to where it should be. Using two cupped hands can illustrate this explanation very clearly.

The patient should then be examined in a supine position with her knees bent up and abducted laterally. The presence of any cystocele

(a) Levator ani muscles
viewed from below

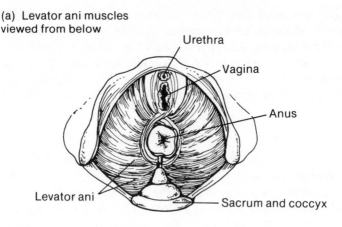

(b) Side view

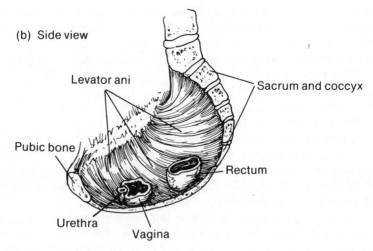

Figure 6.8 *Muscles of the pelvic floor.*

(prolapse of the anterior vaginal wall) or rectocele (prolapse of the posterior vaginal wall) should be noted. If either of these is severe, or if the uterus itself is descending down the vagina, the chances of success from these exercises is probably diminished. They may still be worth a try, especially if the patient is keen. Even if surgery is eventually necessary they will improve the tone and blood-flow locally, thus improving post-operative healing.

The instructor should insert two fingers into the vagina and instruct the patient to squeeze. Many women cannot do so, or do something else such as bear down or contract the buttocks or abdominal muscles. The muscle tone should be carefully assessed, and ideally the examiner should persist until the patient is able to identify the correct action, or at least stop using the wrong muscles. A gentle squeeze will be felt about two finger-joints inside the introitus. It may be useful to ask the patient to imagine that she is attempting to control severe diarrhoea in public in order to locate the muscle. Some women can distinguish a contraction of the anterior portion of the pelvic floor (around the urethra and vagina) from a posterior contraction (around the anus) and can exercise either separately. If this is so, the patient can concentrate her efforts anteriorly. However, this is beyond most women, who are best advised to contract the entire pelvic floor during these exercises.

The exercise programme involves interrupting micturition mid-stream at every opportunity, and practising the same action regularly. Interruption midstream both uses the muscles very effectively and helps to identify what pelvic floor contraction feels like. The patient is instructed to sit on the lavatory with her knees apart, to start passing urine and then, once the stream is coming fast, to stop as quickly and completely as possible. At first she may only be able to slow rather than stop the stream, but that will come with practice. When stopping she should concentrate on the feeling produced – which is the pelvic floor contraction. The bladder should then be emptied completely. Two or three interruptions may be possible per void if the bladder is very full.

Once the pelvic floor has been correctly identified, either by digital examination or by interruption of the urinary stream, the exercises can start in earnest. The patient is instructed to lie, sit, or stand with her knees slightly apart, and slowly but firmly to contract the pelvic floor, to hold it contracted for five seconds, and then to relax. This should be done five times every hour throughout the day. And *every* day! This may sound like a lot at first, but it should be emphasised that the exercises really involve minimal disruption of activities – they can be done almost anywhere without anyone else knowing. They will do no good if practised much less often, but should not be done much more frequently either, as the muscle will become fatigued and ache, and the patient will then be disinclined to continue. If an hourly programme is difficult to remember, the patient can link her exercises to regular daily activities (e.g. brushing her teeth, taking morning coffee, and so on).

Some women like to check they are doing the exercises correctly by inserting a finger into the vagina while exercising, perhaps once a day. They should be able to feel the gentle squeeze for themselves. A useful feedback gadget is the perineometer. This comprises a vaginal probe with a gauge to indicate the strength of squeeze (Figure 6.9). This can tell the patient both that she is exercising correctly and that her muscle power is increasing gradually. This is very important in the phase before symptoms actually improve: it is always tempting to give up unless progress is evident.

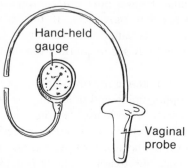

Figure 6.9 *The perineometer.*

It is important after teaching these exercises to see the patient regularly and to re-examine her. This will check that she is using the correct muscles, give her encouragement, and help motivation. It also provides an opportunity to discuss any worries or questions. Usually patients should be seen every two to four weeks. Few will notice any great benefit for six to eight weeks. Most will have improved somewhat by three months if they are going to, although some take six to nine months to achieve maximum benefit from the exercises. It can be difficult to keep the patient doing the exercises consistently for as long as this, although many women do find it becomes an automatic habit.

It is likely that if patients are carefully selected – i.e. mild to moderate stress incontinence, without significant prolapse in a motivated woman – over 80% can achieve a cure using pelvic-floor exercises. The patient can often thus avoid surgery and have the satisfaction of having cured herself. As an added benefit, many find that their own, and their partner's, sexual enjoyment is increased as muscle tone improves.

Physiotherapists may use electrical stimulation as an aid to pelvic floor exercises. Vaginal faradism uses a vaginal probe which electrically induces a pelvic floor contraction. This may be useful in helping a patient who is totally unable to do this voluntarily to identify the correct sensation, and thus know what to aim for. Neither faradism nor interferential therapy have any proven value in treatment programmes and are no more effective than exercises alone, provided that these are properly taught and monitored.

Surgery for stress incontinence

Women with a moderate degree of stress incontinence which has not responded to the above exercises, and those with a severe problem, especially if associated with considerable prolapse, often require surgery to alleviate their condition. The choice of operation will depend on the individual surgeon's expertise and the patient's preference.

Vaginal repair. There are a great many variations upon vaginal repair. Usually the anterior vaginal wall is divided to display the bladder neck and proximal urethra. These are mobilised upwards and held up with buttress sutures. A vaginal hysterectomy, amputation of the cervix, or posterior vaginal wall repair may be performed at the same time, if indicated.

Sling procedures. The alternative approach is via an abdominal, usually 'bikini-line', incision. Either organic (strips of fascia) or synthetic material (e.g. polypropylene or polyethylene) is used to support and elevate the bladder neck by attachment to ligaments or periosteum. The Aldridge Sling, Marshall-Marchetti-Krantz and Colposuspension are the most widely practised operations.

As with any operation, there is a slight risk attached to these procedures. The vaginal repair has the advantages that it is not a major procedure, there is no abdominal scar, and rehabilitation is rapid, with usually only five to seven days in hospital. Unfortunately success rates vary, and while they are excellent in experienced hands, they may be under 50% in others (Stanton, 1977). Conversely a sling procedure is a more major operation, involves an abdominal incision, and up to two weeks in hospital. Overall success rates are higher than for vaginal surgery, especially in the long term. Fewer surgeons are experienced with suprapubic than with vaginal procedures.

Any type of surgery requires careful pre- and post-operative counselling. This can increase both the success of the procedure and the patient's satisfaction and adjustment. The patient must be given a full explanation of the procedure and what to expect. If hysterectomy is likely to be necessary, this is a decision which involves careful thought and discussion with spouse or family. It should be made clear that none of these operations can guarantee success, and the chances of cure should be honestly discussed. Patients who are led to unrealistic expectations of total cure tend to be highly intolerant and disappointed if any symptoms, however mild, persist post-operatively.

If the patient has not yet completed her family, surgery should usually be delayed until after the final pregnancy, especially with sling operations, as vaginal delivery might both be difficult and undo the effects of the surgery. Every patient should be warned that there is a possibility of stress incontinence recurring at a later date. This is especially true if she undertakes vigorous exercise or heavy lifting. Women who only leak when they lift heavy weights, or have a heavy manual job, should probably be discouraged from opting for surgery. As the convalescent periods are different (a few weeks for vaginal procedures, up to three months for slings), women with heavy family or career commitments may prefer the former, even in the knowledge that success rates are lower.

Post-operative advice should involve instructions to take things easy for the convalescent period, and especially to avoid lifting and abdominal effort. The patient should also refrain from sexual intercourse for six weeks to allow full healing. Many women experience problems in returning to an active and fulfilling sex life after surgery. Sometimes the reason for this is psychological, because of a changed body image, especially after an hysterectomy. There may be physical discomfort because of incomplete healing or local infection. More commonly the actual anatomy of the vagina is altered, and it often takes both partners a while to adjust to the new, smaller contours. Sometimes there is a ridge or kink in the vaginal wall. The woman may also be nervous or anxious in case it should hurt, or the operation might be 'undone', and so be understimulated and poorly lubricated. Sometimes simple explanations, reassurance that no harm can be done, and possibly a tube of KY Jelly for lubrication, will resolve the problem. (The lubricant can be made considerably pleasanter and more acceptable to use by warming the tube in a bowl of warm water before application.) Occasionally it may be advisable to experiment with new positions for intercourse to overcome problems with a taut anterior vaginal wall.

In the past many women have undergone multiple operations for stress incontinence, which has either been unaffected or recurred. Sometimes this was because the original diagnosis was wrong, and the woman really had detrusor instability rather than geniune stress incontinence. Hopefully the increased use of urodynamic facilities will help to avoid this in the future. The first operation has the highest chance of success. As more urologists and gynaecologists become interested and expert in incontinence surgery, and as understanding of the mechanism of successful operations increases, it is to be hoped that there will be fewer failures.

Neo-urethra. In a few specialist centres a technique has been developed for the construction of a completely new urethra for the female from a flap of bladder muscle. This may be used for those with congenital abnormalities, or those with a urethra rendered scarred and function-less by repeated surgery. It is too early to evaluate the success of this procedure, but it may hold out hope for the future.

URINARY FISTULA

A fistula or 'false passage' between the bladder and vagina will cause continuous, uncontrollable, passive incontinence. It is relatively uncommon in Western countries, where it is mostly caused iatrogen-ically as a result of a mishap during gynaecological surgery or after pelvic irradiation for tumour. It is more common in underdeveloped countries as a complication of obstructed delivery. Prolonged pressure of the baby's head causes tissue necrosis, and the resultant sloughing leaves a fistula.

Fistulae caused surgically or during childbirth are usually repaired surgically. This is done vaginally six to ten weeks after the trauma, provided that the patient is in good health. Post-irradiation fistulae are often far more difficult to repair, as there is usually much scar tissue and an avascular zone in the vagina. The patient is often also in poor health.

There can be little doubt about the misery occasioned by a urinary fistula. The constant leakage of urine is extremely difficult to cope with, and there is no pad yet available that will cope totally reliably with this degree of female incontinence. Quality of life often becomes very poor, and the patient becomes isolated and depressed. There is no respite, waking or sleeping. Where the defect cannot be closed surgically, a urinary diversion into an ileal conduit (see Chapter 4) is strongly recommended, wherever the patient is fit enough. Even though a stoma means continuous 'incontinence', this is at least controllable with a suitable collection bag. If the patient is too unwell for this major surgery or does not want it, the best that can be offered at present is one of the largest body-worn pads (see Chapter 13). These will need to be supplied freely in large quantities.

INCONTINENCE AND SEXUAL ACTIVITY

Some women experience urinary incontinence during sexual activity. It is not known how common this is, but certainly any nurse working in an incontinence clinic will encounter it quite often. It may be difficult for a patient to talk about this problem, and the nurse should provide an opportunity and give appropriate prompts to make such a discussion possible. Most women also have bladder symptoms at other times, but for a few this is the only occasion they experience incontinence. Either way, it can be a source of considerable worry and embarrassment. The patient may not have openly discussed the leakage with her partner. Other couples accept it as a minor nuisance which can be laughed about together.

Leakage most usually occurs during intercourse or at orgasm (often the entire bladder contents are emptied at orgasm). The mechanism for this incontinence is unknown – hardly surprisingly, it is difficult to investigate. It is likely that mechanical pressure or a detrusor contraction underlie the problem. Sometimes treatment for a known bladder dysfunction (for example drug therapy for detrusor instability) will cure the incontinence. Otherwise the patient needs plenty of reassurance that the symptom is of no pathological significance, as well as advice on learning to live with it. The patient should, when it is possible and appropriate, empty the bladder as fully as possible before commencing sexual activity. The bed or other surface can be protected with a thick towel or washable drawsheet (see Chapter 13) to minimise discomfort and inconvenience afterwards. For couples with a close and sympathetic relationship a post-coital bath or shower together is often the only consequence of the woman's bladder problem.

INCONTINENCE IN PREGNANCY

Incontinence of urine is a common symptom in pregnancy. Probably over one-half of all primiparous women and over three-quarters of multiparous women experience some incontinence. The majority complain of increased frequency of micturition, usually starting in the first trimester and persisting until the birth. Various possible causes have been proposed for this frequency, including polydipsia, mechanical pressure on the bladder, and the onset of an unstable bladder. None of these really explains this frequency adequately, but each may be true for some women. Most expect frequency, and few are unduly incapacitated by it.

Incontinence during pregnancy is usually experienced as stress incontinence. Sometimes this has been present prior to pregnancy, but for many it is new. It is seldom severe enough to represent a significant problem. This is obviously a good time for women to be taught pelvic floor exercises. Many women find that it disappears after the delivery of the baby. Stress incontinence as a new problem is quite rare immediately after childbirth.

Most women are unsurprised by some incontinence during pregnancy. It is very important that the midwife, health visitor and physiotherapist work together to teach women about the functioning of the pelvic floor muscles, and how to look after and strengthen their vulnerable sphincter mechanism.

OCCLUSIVE DEVICES

Several devices are available which control female urinary incontinence by occluding the urethra mechanically. Although they are most appropriate for women with stress incontinence, they may be used to control any type of leakage. The aim is to restore normal pressure and anatomical relationships by lifting and supporting the bladder neck and urethra. They do not treat the problem, so should seldom be the first choice of therapy except where the woman is unfit for treatment, or does not want it.

Tampons. Some women find that a large menstrual tampon worn in the vagina will control mild incontinence. This is particularly suitable for women who are accustomed to using tampons and have only an occasional problem. For example, a woman who leaks slightly while playing sport may choose this method to control leakage. Anyone who says her incontinence is better during a period should be questioned about her method of sanitary protection, as wearing a tampon may be the reason for improvement. She will then trust this method of control.

It is unwise to wear tampons continuously; because of their

absorbent properties they tend to make the vagina sore and very dry. Some women use a home-made foam-rubber tampon instead. This tends to be softer, and so somewhat less effective, but avoids some of the dryness. Rocket Ltd make a foam pessary with a withdrawal string in three sizes. These can be washed and re-used if desired (Figure 6.10).

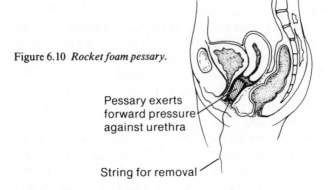

Figure 6.10 *Rocket foam pessary.*

Pessary exerts
forward pressure
against urethra

String for removal

Ring pessary (Figure 6.11). Where stress incontinence is associated with an obvious prolapse of the anterior vaginal wall, a ring pessary may be fitted by a gynaecologist. The rings come in a wide range of sizes and are made from PVC. Insertion is usually momentarily uncomfortable, but once in situ they are generally comfortable if the correct size is chosen. The ring is indwelling and needs to be changed every three to six months.

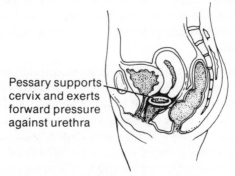

Pessary supports
cervix and exerts
forward pressure
against urethra

Figure 6.11 *Ring pessary. The ring stays in place, as shown here, supported by the bone and ligaments of the pelvic rim.*

Careful explanation is needed before the pessary is inserted. Some women dislike the idea and reject it. It should be carefully established that the patient is not still sexually active, as a ring pessary is then obviously unsuitable. Some older women with genital atrophy, and some nulliparous women have an introitus too small to allow one to be inserted.

The ring pessary is most suited to the older woman with stress incontinence who fails to respond to pelvic-floor exercises and does not want or is unfit for surgery. Mental and physical disability are no contra-indication, as once in situ no further management is needed by patient or carer.

Bonnar device (Figure 6.12). This is an inflatable silicone device which fits into the vagina. The two 'horns' should sit in the lateral fornices on either side of the cervix, and the balloon is inflated to support the bladder neck. The small hand-pump is reversed to deflate the balloon for micturition. The device is inserted by the user, and should be removed and washed at least once daily.

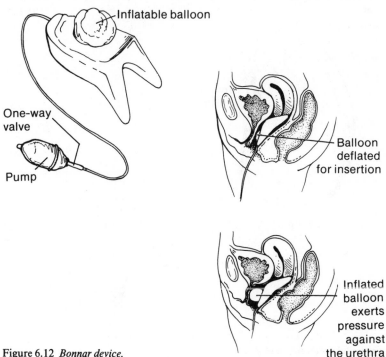

Figure 6.12 *Bonnar device.*

This device is only suitable for women with considerable manual dexterity. As only one size is available some find it too large to insert, while others find it falls out. Women with a moderate degree of prolapse also have difficulty retaining it in place. A few find it is uncomfortable in use.

Edwards device (Figure 6.13). This is a pubo-vaginal spring made from rigid perspex with a metal spring. The triangle fits over the pubic bone and the spring is adjusted to exert pressure anteriorly to the vaginal wall. As with the Bonnar device, manual dexterity is essential. Three sizes are available. It must be removed for micturition.

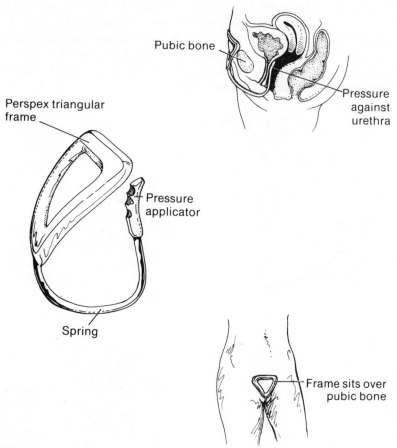

Figure 6.13 *Edwards device.*

Female Incontinence

Except for the tampon, all these devices should only be used with medical or nursing supervision. The latter two in particular may cause pressure problems, especially if the user has diminished sensation. In practice only a minority of women find them acceptable, usable and of benefit. None of the devices has a high success rate in controlling incontinence, and many women dislike the idea anyway. However, they do work for some women, and should be borne in mind as an option in management.

REFERENCES AND FURTHER READING

Harrison, S., 1975. 'Physiotherapy in the treatment of stress incontinence'. *Nursing Mirror*, 141, 2, 52–53.

Mandelstam, D., 1978. 'The pelvic floor'. *Physiotherapy*, 64, 8, 236–239.

Montgomery, E., 1983. *Regaining Bladder Control*. John Wright, Bristol.

Stanton, S. L., 1977. *Female Urinary Incontinence*. Lloyd-Luke, London.

Stanton, S. L., (ed.), 1978. 'Clinics in obstetrics and gynaecology'. *Gynaecological Urology*, 5, 1.

Stanton, S. L., Tanagho, E. A., 1980. *Surgery of Female Incontinence*. Springer-Verlag, Berlin.

Stanton, S. L., 1984. *Clinical Gynaecologic Urology*. C. V. Mosby, St. Louis.

127

Chapter 7

Male Incontinence

While men can suffer incontinence for reasons outlined elsewhere in this book, certain problems affect the male exclusively and are dealt with separately in this chapter. Men seem to be especially reluctant to seek help for incontinence, which is often thought of as a 'woman's problem', and the nurse may be the first person the patient confides in.

PROSTATIC HYPERTROPHY

From the fourth decade of life onwards all men have some degree of benign enlargement of the prostate gland (Figure 7.1). About one man in ten will experience symptoms.

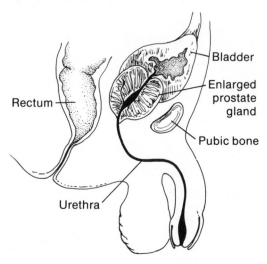

Figure 7.1 *Prostatic hypertrophy.*

Symptoms

Symptoms caused by an enlarged prostate gland relate mostly to the outflow obstruction that this causes. Hesitancy, a slow, weak urinary stream, and terminal dribbling at the end of micturition are common. Often the bladder does not empty completely and chronic residual urine is present. This may cause frequency and nocturia (indeed, nocturia is very often the first symptom noticed by the patient), with dysuria if the residual urine becomes infected. Urgency with urge incontinence or an almost continual dribbling overflow incontinence may be present. Sometimes rectal symptoms are troublesome – either a continuous desire to defaecate caused by prostate pressure on the rectum, or haemorrhoids resulting from repeated straining to micturate. On other occasions the first symptom the patient experiences is acute retention of urine.

Signs

The nurse may be the first person to spot the tense, distended abdomen of an elderly man who is totally unaware that his bladder is full to overflowing. If infection is superimposed, the urine may become cloudy and foul-smelling, occasionally with haematuria. A large residual volume may obstruct ureteric outflow with consequent back pressure to the kidneys and the development of hydronephrosis. If this is the case, the patient may be confused, with anorexia, weight loss, anaemia and dehydration resulting from uraemia.

Often by the time help is sought the problem has been present for many years. If the detrusor muscle is repeatedly trying to overcome raised outflow resistance, the muscle tends to hypertrophy and may develop a secondary detrusor instability and trabeculation (weakened outpouchings between hypertrophied muscle bundles).

Investigation

A careful history will elicit many of the above symptoms, which are often aggravated by cold weather or alcohol. It is especially important to distinguish between symptoms of prostatism and those of a pure detrusor instability (instability more often presents as frequency, urgency, urge incontinence, with little or no voiding difficulty). Examination digitally per rectum may reveal an enlarged prostate gland, although in fact the palpable size of the gland bears no direct relationship to the degree of outflow obstruction. Indeed, even a minimally enlarged prostate can obstruct the urethra, while some very large glands cause no problems. Abdominal examination may enable palpation of the bladder, or alternatively a faecal impaction which may mimic prostatism. The perineal skin may be sore or excoriated because of urinary incontinence, but not all men with prostatic enlargement are incontinent.

A free flow-rate (see Chapter 3) will usually reveal a low, prolonged flow, sometimes interrupted or with a very long 'tail'. A residual catheterisation post-micturition may prove difficult if the prostate is very large or if insufficient anaesthetic gel is used. Often a large volume of residual urine is present. A midstream urine specimen and blood tests (for renal function) should be routine, and an intravenous pyelogram will be performed if renal impairment is suspected. A cystometrogram, if performed, will show a high voiding pressure with a low flow-rate and often a detrusor instability during filling. Many prostatectomies are performed without prior cystometrogram, but if the diagnosis of an unstable bladder is suspected the test is essential. A prostatectomy performed on a man with an unobstructed urethra and an unstable bladder will merely reduce his outflow resistance and make him even more likely to be incontinent.

PROSTATECTOMY

Roughly one-half of men who experience symptoms from prostate enlargement eventually require a prostatectomy. At present there is no non-surgical alternative for men whose life is made miserable by recurrent infections or incontinence, or whose health is endangered by renal damage. Unfortunately, the waiting lists for this type of surgery are often very long, and much unnecessary misery results. There are two alternative surgical approaches commonly used to remove the prostate.

Transurethral resection of the prostate (TUR or TURP)
A transurethral resection of the prostate is performed via a specially adapted cystoscope, and is a relatively safe operation. As no abdominal wound is involved, patients can mobilise comfortably very soon after surgery (this is important in older patients). All but the largest prostates can be removed transurethrally, but removal must be done by an experienced surgeon as it is possible to damage the external urethral sphincter, which will almost always result in incontinence (see below).

130

Retropubic prostatectomy (RPP)
A retropubic prostatectomy is performed via a lower abdominal incision and the prostate is 'shelled out' of its capsule. This is in many ways a simpler operation requiring less skill than a TURP, and it can be performed for even the largest prostates. However, it does involve an abdominal wound and probably a higher risk of morbidity and mortality. Mobilisation may be delayed by abdominal discomfort, and the length of hospital stay is double that for TURP.

Complications of prostatectomy
As with any general anaesthetic a certain risk of mortality and morbidity is involved, especially in the older age-groups. Some centres now use an epidural anaesthetic in those unfit for, or especially at risk from, a general anaesthetic.

Incontinence is dealt with separately below.

Impotence is quite common following prostatectomy. About 7% of previously potent men will be rendered partially or totally impotent. If previous erectile problems were experienced, at least 30% will be worsened post-operatively. The majority of men are infertile following prostatectomy because of retrograde ejaculation of semen into the bladder. A small number (2%–3%) develop a post-operative stricture.

Altogether roughly 20% of men experience some complication after such surgery. It is important to discuss these possibilities fully with the patient prior to making a decision about surgery. Unless there are urgent medical indications (e.g. imminent renal failure), the patient should be encouraged to decide whether his symptoms are troublesome enough to warrant the risk of the possible complications. It should not be forgotten that an elderly man may value his fertility and potency as highly as a younger man. Good pre-operative counselling will avoid many later regrets and recriminations.

Having said this, the vast majority of men with symptoms of voiding difficulties or incontinence arising from prostatic hypertrophy will (if correctly diagnosed) benefit from prostatectomy, and much misery is relieved by this simple operation. Many men take these symptoms for granted with advancing age and suffer unnecessarily. There is already a need for urodynamic clinics and urological surgeons to be more widely available to cope with present problems, let alone the likely increased demands of an increasing aged population.

CARCINOMA OF THE PROSTATE

With advancing age the likelihood of malignant changes in the prostate increases. By the ninth decade 80% of men have a prostatic carcinoma. In the very elderly this is a relatively 'benign', localised condition but it can become invasive and metastatic in younger men. The symptoms are identical with those of benign prostatic hypertrophy in 80% of cases, and for this reason alone it is worth investigating any man with symptoms of prostatism. The gland may feel hard on rectal examination but the only sure method of diagnosis is by cystoscopic biopsy of the gland.

URETHRAL STRICTURE

Although urethral strictures may present in women, they are uncommon, and most occur in males. A stricture, or narrowing of the urethra, results from scarred healing after an infection (urethritis) or trauma. Figure 7.2 shows the common sites for stricture. At the external meatus it may be caused by instrumentation, especially an indwelling catheter. At the peno-scrotal junction a catheter can cause pressure necrosis and subsequent stricture. A stricture may extend

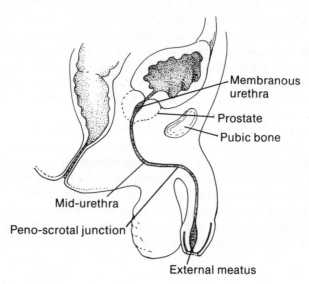

Figure 7.2 *Common sites of urethral stricture.*

along the length of the midurethra following a gonococcal infection. A ruptured membranous urethra will often heal as a stricture.

Symptoms are usually similar to prostatism: voiding difficulty, possibly with overflow incontinence and renal problems. Often a possible causative agent can be identified in the patient's history (e.g. catheterisation following major surgery or a previous urethritis). The diagnosis is made either on classical difficulty passing a catheter, or on micturating cystogram or cystoscopy.

Treatment of a stricture involves either regular dilatation (usually under local anaesthetic using graduated bougies) or surgical division of the stricture (internal urethrotomy). With both of these methods the symptoms may recur.

BLADDER-NECK OBSTRUCTION

Bladder-neck obstruction results from fibrous, muscular or glandular hypertrophy of the bladder neck. It is most commonly seen secondarily to a neuropathic lesion of the bladder or to chronic prostatitis. The symptoms are, again, very similar to those arising from an enlarged prostate (voiding difficulties, with possible residual urine, overflow incontinence, and renal impairment). Classically a bladder-neck obstruction presents at an earlier age than prostatism, and the prostate is seldom enlarged. Treatment is either to attempt to relax the obstruction pharmacologically (e.g. phenoxybenzamine 5mg t.d.s.) or to surgically incise or resect the bladder neck. The surgical approach carries a slight risk of causing an incontinence not previously present.

POST-MICTURITION DRIBBLING

In some men incontinence takes the form of post-micturition dribbling. A small amount of urine is passed, usually without much sensation, up to several minutes after micturition is completed. This should be distinguished from terminal dribbling, which is a very slow dribbling stream at the end of the act of micturition. If clothing has been replaced the dribble, although often only a few millilitres of urine, may be enough to soak through underpants and trousers and to leave an embarrassing wet patch, especially if trousers are lightweight or pale in colour.

Most commonly a post-micturition dribble is caused by pooling of urine in the bulbar urethra (Figure 7.3(a)). The reason for this abnormally lax and wide bulb is unknown. If the diagnosis is in doubt a micturating cystogram will clearly show this pool in the bulbar urethra after micturition. A simple explanation of the cause, reassurance that the problem has no significance, and instruction on emptying the urine will usually solve the problem. The patient is instructed to express the urine by firm upward and forward pressure by fingers or fist behind the scrotum at the end of micturition. The trapped urine will be milked out (Figure 7.3(b)).

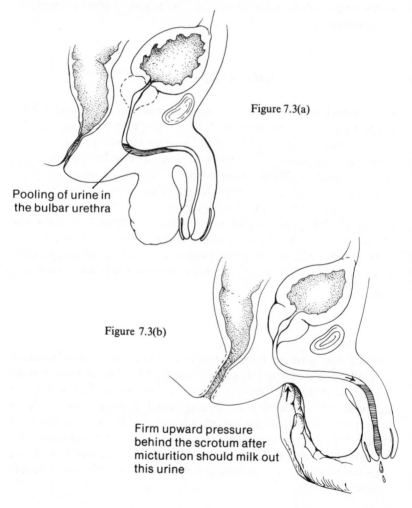

Figure 7.3(a)

Pooling of urine in the bulbar urethra

Figure 7.3(b)

Firm upward pressure behind the scrotum after micturition should milk out this urine

Post-micturition dribble may also occur in men with prostatic enlargement, with an unstable bladder (sometimes a powerful 'after contraction' forces out a few extra drops), or with an atonic bladder. In all of these conditions other symptoms usually co-exist and suggest the cause. The man with simple pooling in the bulbar urethra will seldom have any other micturition problems.

If the problem is persistent a dribble pouch (see Chapter 13) may contain the leakage.

POST-PROSTATECTOMY INCONTINENCE

Many men experience increased urgency and slight incontinence immediately after prostatectomy. It should be explained that time is necessary to adjust to the new weaker outflow resistance and that it should settle within a few weeks. Pelvic floor exercises are very useful at this time. The patient is instructed to interrupt micturition midstream at every void. At first he may only be able to slow rather than stop the stream. At the same time a regime of regular pelvic floor contractions is also taught – the patient is instructed to contract the pelvic floor muscles five times per hour throughout the day. On a surgical ward with several prostatectomy patients this soon becomes part of the routine. The exercises can considerably strengthen the pelvic floor supports to the external sphincter, on which the patient is now reliant for continence. They also rapidly increase confidence in the ability to control any incontinence.

Those patients who had an unstable bladder prior to prostatectomy will take rather longer to regain continence post-operatively. Instability secondary to long-standing obstruction will not disappear immediately, and it can take six to twelve months for the detrusor muscle to adjust to the new, lower outflow resistance. For a few men the instability is persistent and troublesome, causing frequency, urgency and urge incontinence. In most cases this will respond to standard therapy for unstable bladders (usually drugs and bladder training – see Chapter 4). Explanation and reassurance and the provision of a suitable incontinence aid, while needed, will help to tide the patient over this distressing post-operative phase. Few things are more depressing to the patient than an operation which leaves his symptoms unchanged or worsened. If the patient knows this is to be expected and will improve, he will often cope much better.

In a few instances post-prostatectomy incontinence results from inadvertent sphincter damage at operation. This is more likely after

TURP than RPP. If sphincter damage has been extensive, pelvic floor exercises will seldom effect a cure. For these men the only hope of continence is further surgery. Three different implantable devices may be used to correct this type of incontinence (or that caused by sphincter damage from any other source).

Kaufman urinary incontinence prosthesis (Figure 7.4(a))
The Kaufman device is the simplest of the three implantable devices. It consists of a silicone gel prosthesis covered with open-cell foam (to allow tissue ingrowth) and two dacron velour straps. The device is surgically implanted over the urethral bulb and the straps wrapped around the urethra and tied. The pressure exerted by the flexible prosthesis on the urethra should raise urethral closure pressure sufficiently to restore continence. If necessary, the prosthesis can be further inflated post-operatively via a perineal injection.

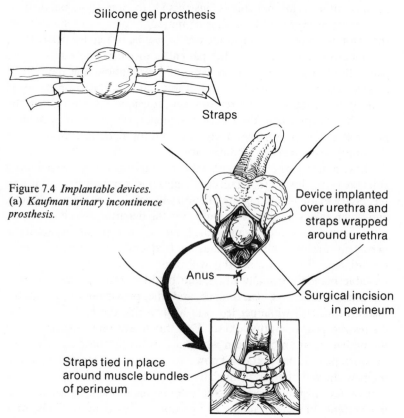

Silicone gel prosthesis

Straps

Figure 7.4 *Implantable devices.*
(a) *Kaufman urinary incontinence prosthesis.*

Device implanted over urethra and straps wrapped around urethra

Anus

Surgical incision in perineum

Straps tied in place around muscle bundles of perineum

Rosen prosthesis (Figure 7.4(b))

The Rosen prosthesis is made from silicone elastomer. It has two arms which position over the urethra and an inflatable balloon opposing them. As with the Kaufman, the device is implanted surgically via the perineum. A reservoir of saline is implanted in the scrotum. A valve proximal to this reservoir is squeezed to allow micturition by deflating the balloon. After micturition the reservoir is squeezed to re-inflate the balloon and re-establish continence. Unlike the Kaufman, which requires no manipulation once in place, the Rosen device requires the patient to have considerable manual dexterity and mental alertness. The patient with diminished bladder awareness will need to release the valve regularly by the clock.

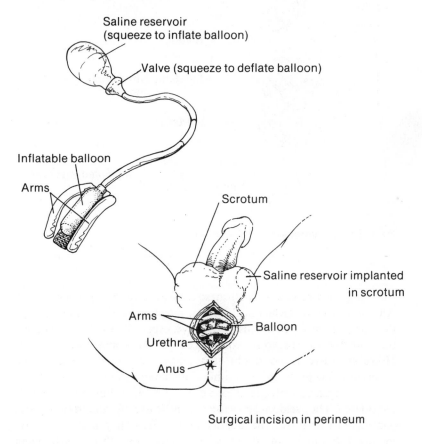

Figure 7.4 (b) *Rosen prosthesis.*

Brantley-Scott artificial sphincter

This device employs an inflated cuff around the urethra and a reservoir which is squeezed to deflate the cuff (Figure 7.4(c)). It can be used in women as well as men, in which case the reservoir is implanted in the labia rather than the scrotum. Considerable improvements have been made in the design of this device in recent years and the current model appears to function well.

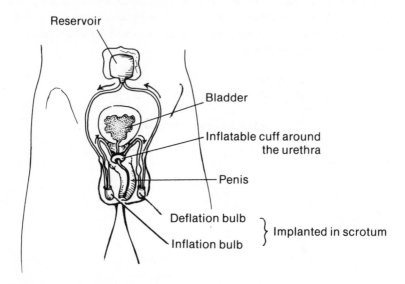

Figure 7.4 (c) *Brantley-Scott artificial sphincter.*

The long-term results with all these devices have yet to be evaluated. All carry risks of mechanical failure, rejection, and erosion through the body's tissues. All are also expensive, especially the latter two, and the number of surgeons experienced in their insertion is small. However, there is no doubt that many patients do benefit, and experience few problems. Certainly if the alternative is a lifetime's use of aids or a urinary diversion, one of these devices should be seriously considered. They seldom leave the patient worse off, and in most cases considerably improve the quality of his life. They may even save money in the long run, and it is to be hoped that their development will continue and that they become more widely available.

CONTROL OF INCONTINENCE: THE PENILE CLAMP

The penile clamp aims to control incontinence by external mechanical occlusion of the penile urethra. The most commonly used is the Cunningham clamp (Eschmann, Figure 7.5). The foam-lined metal arms fit across the penis laterally and close on a ratchet until incontinence is controlled. It is available in three sizes.

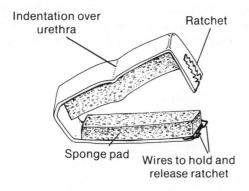

Figure 7.5 *Penile clamp.*

The penile clamp should be used with extreme caution as it can cause considerable damage, even pressure necrosis, to the penis. Each clamp must be individually fitted and moulded by an expert. At the first fitting it should be left in situ for very short periods only, and inspected every few minutes to check for oedema, inflammation, or cyanosis to the penis. Some men find the device too uncomfortable or heavy to use, especially if it has to be closed very tightly to control incontinence. It is inadvisable to use the clamp with men who have high-pressure unstable bladders, as the contractions are then against greater resistance and the instability may be exacerbated, the bladder neck damaged, and vesico-ureteric reflux may even occur.

To use a penile clamp the patient must have good manual dexterity and be sufficiently mentally able to appreciate both how to use it and the dangers of improper use. It can seldom be used if the penis is retracted. The patient should be given very clear instructions on using the clamp, and how to position it, and be told to stop using it immediately if sores, oedema, or cyanosis develop.

The penile clamp should really be seen as a last resort when all else has failed to control incontinence. It does have uses which cannot be fulfilled by any of the aids outlined in Chapter 13. For example, the incontinent sportsman cannot compete in a leg bag but may be able to disguise a clamp under his shorts. The sexually active man may wish to remove his penile sheath adhesive and have a wash prior to intercourse, and use the clamp in the interim. Some men regularly use a clamp very successfully, and often this is considerably more convenient than wearing a collecting bag all the time – the bladder is simply used as a reservoir and the clamp released at appropriate intervals. A penile clamp should never be handed out as the first line of management for incontinence in the male, but if fitted properly and given with adequate instruction it can be successful in restoring the patient to continence.

Chapter 8

Incontinence in the Elderly

Incontinence becomes more common as one gets older. However, incontinence is not an inevitable part of growing old, as evidenced by the fact that most old people are continent. Unfortunately, incontinence does tend to be accepted far more readily in old age, by sufferer and professionals alike, so it is much less likely to receive systematic investigation or treatment than the same symptoms in a younger person. It is common for the elderly to be told: 'It's just old age', or 'What do you expect at your age?'

It is not intended, by devoting a separate chapter to incontinence and the elderly, to imply that they should be treated differently from younger incontinent people. All the causes, investigations and treatment referred to elsewhere in this volume are equally relevant to the aged, and the same methods apply. This chapter merely highlights certain additional age-related problems which may influence continence.

Surveys of incontinence have yielded widely different prevalence figures. Probably about 10% of people over sixty-five have some degree of incontinence if they live in the community. This figure rises to between 20% and 40% among those in institutional care. As with younger age-groups, women are more likely to suffer than men, although the disparity tends to lessen with time (especially after the age of seventy-five).

For many old people, their incontinence is not a new, or even recent, problem. Some will have hidden it for years or decades, and are only forced to reveal it when they require medical or nursing attention for some other disorder. Many learn to cope in their own way, but for others it causes a very severe disruption to their lives. At the very least they may be uncomfortable and ashamed. At worst they may eventually fail to cope independently at home, and either become a burden to relatives or friends or need permanent alternative care. Many relatives do manage to look after severely incontinent old people in the community and tolerate a considerable workload and

141

disruption. Symptoms which tend to be less well tolerated are faecal incontinence, persistent disturbances at night, and incontinence in an opposite-sexed parent (Sanford, 1975). These, more commonly than urinary incontinence alone, may lead to requests for institutional care. Once an elderly person is in need of long-term care he is much more likely to end up in hospital than in a home if he is incontinent.

Britain has a population which will contain an increasing proportion of old people over the next decades. The proportion of the very elderly is increasing even more rapidly. In order to ensure that as many as possible of the elderly are able to live independent lives in the community, with a high quality of life, one of the most important factors will be effective diagnosis, treatment and management facilities for those with bladder or bowel dysfunction. Much more attention must be focused on ways of preventing incontinence. A change of attitude among those working with and caring for old people is necessary in many instances. The promotion of continence should be a priority. As the elderly are the group of sufferers least likely to seek help, facilities should be geared to providing prompt practical help involving a minimum of effort and embarrassment, and services should be widely advertised.

'VICTORIAN DECENCY'

Most of those whom we now classify as 'elderly' were born in or near the Victorian era, with its strict sense of morality and decency. A society which covered up table legs because they were considered 'suggestive' also discouraged all mention of bodily functions, particularly elimination. The water closet, or 'W.C.', was usually outside the house, even at the bottom of the garden, and certainly well away from the polite environment of the parlour. As a result, many old people are extremely ignorant about the way their bodies work, especially their excretory and reproductive organs. Often they have no words to describe micturition or defaecation, except maybe childish words which they may be reluctant to use if they recognise them as inappropriate to adults. Thus even starting to talk to an old person about incontinence can be difficult until a mutually understood vocabulary has been established. The nurse must always be certain that she and the patient mean the same thing, whatever words are used. It is all too easy to upset and alienate a patient by using jargon which the professional takes for granted, but which may be unclear or even misleading to the lay person.

'Incontinence' has had several other meanings than the one used in this book. It was often used in 19th century literature to mean 'without any apparent control' (as in 'he rushed incontinently from the room' or 'he talked incontinently about . . .'). The term has also been used to denote lack of moral self-control, or sexual promiscuity. The Oxford English Dictionary lists 'wanting in self-restraint, especially in regard to sexual appetite' before 'unable to keep something in, of secrets, tongue, urine', even today. Many elderly people see 'incontinent' as a prejudicial label, implying moral degeneracy, or at least that the individual is in some way to blame for the condition. Most wish to avoid the label 'incontinent' at all costs, and would use it only for those people who are totally unable to hold any urine, or who wet openly in public without any apparent compunction. Many fear reaching this state, and comments such as 'I wet myself and I'm worried I might become incontinent' will be familiar to many nurses.

Passing urine or faeces is something which most elderly people, particularly women, have always done behind a closed, locked door. Shyness often exists, even between couples who have been married for many years. Unwillingness to talk about problems with a spouse present should be recognised and respected. Yet many old people are expected to pass urine or faeces in surroundings that are far from private. A commode in the bedroom or living-room is often suggested for those with urgency and poor mobility, without it being discovered that the patient would rather be wet than be seen (or heard) passing urine by a husband or wife. In hospital, lack of privacy can have an extremely inhibiting effect on bowel or bladder emptying. Curtains may hide the sight, but do not disguise the sound, smell, and knowledge of what is going on behind them. A nurse hovering outside (or even inside) the lavatory door likewise makes elimination difficult and often incomplete. Some people are even embarrassed if asked within earshot of others whether they would like toilet facilities: they would rather refuse than let everyone know where they are going.

Elderly people often have very individualistic habits or rituals relating to elimination. Many are extremely fastidious about personal hygiene and always have a thorough wash after a bowel action, and are meticulous about handwashing after every visit to the lavatory. Yet it has been found that most nurses are negligent in offering even handwashing facilities to patients. This is especially true if a bedpan or a commode by the bed is used. The patient may consequently become unwilling to use these, especially before meals, and in attempting to hang on, become incontinent.

Some people have been brought up with the myth that it is possible to catch venereal disease or cystitis from public lavatory seats. As a result, they are very reluctant to sit down on ward lavatories, or even to use them at all. This is especially so if facilities are unclean, or shared by both sexes. Others have long-standing rituals for their bowel function and will become constipated if these are broken. Each patient's usual preferences and habits need to be discovered by the nurse (whether at home or in a hospital), and wherever possible facilities should be provided to cater for these needs.

THE PHYSIOLOGICAL EFFECTS OF AGEING ON CONTINENCE

The effects of ageing on bowel function are considered elsewhere (see Chapter 14), so most of the factors described here relate to urinary incontinence.

The ageing kidney

There is a considerable reduction in glomerular filtration rate with advancing age. This is caused by a combination of structural degeneration of the kidney and reduced cardiac output. The ability to rid the body of waste products is therefore decreased. The kidney receives a smaller proportion of cardiac output by day, although this may return to normal at night when the demands of other organs are lessened. This may explain why many elderly people have a disturbed diurnal rhythm of urine production. Young adults produce most urine by day and relatively little when asleep. Older people often produce urine at the same rate day and night, or even produce more at night. (This is most pronounced in the confused and demented, possibly because of their generally disturbed circadian rhythms.) It is one reason why so many elderly people have to get up at night to pass urine, often several times – they are actually producing more urine per night than the bladder can hold.

Urinary tract infection

Infection of the bladder or kidneys is common among the elderly. Significant bacteriuria is present in 20% of women over sixty-five and men over seventy-five living at home (Brocklehurst et al., 1968). In hospital this rises to 30%–40% of long-stay inpatients. The vast majority of these infections are asymptomatic and probably harmless. Most are low-grade and chronic, often associated with voiding difficulties and residual urine (e.g. in prostatic hypertrophy or neurological damage).

It has not been proven that urinary tract infection causes incontinence, nor indeed vice versa. An acute cystitis may precipitate incontinence in someone already at risk, and should therefore be treated. A chronic infection is unlikely to be the cause of incontinence. Failure of therapy or re-infection are common, so if one or two courses of antibiotics fail to clear the infection it should be left alone (Brocklehurst, 1977).

Age changes in the bladder

There is an increased tendency for the bladder to be trabeculated with age as the detrusor muscle hypertrophies and there is a loss of supporting elastic tissue. Fibrosis becomes commoner, possibly as a result of chronic infection, and may result in bladder-neck stenosis and voiding difficulties.

The urethral mucosa may prolapse down through the external urethral meatus, and this can form an ulcerating caruncle. The significance of this is unknown, but it tends to be associated with incontinence. If painful or bleeding, it can be treated with vaginal oestrogens (see below).

As elastic tissue and muscles weaken, stress incontinence becomes commoner in women (see Chapter 6). With atrophy of all pelvic organs the urethral meatus may recede along the vaginal wall, out of sight. This causes great difficulty if a catheter is to be passed, and the woman may have to be catheterised in a lateral position from behind with flexed knees.

All the bladder dysfunctions which can cause incontinence become commoner in old age. It is also far more likely that the elderly incontinent person will have more than one bladder abnormality, such as an unstable bladder and stress incontinence, or a voiding problem with unstable contractions. This means that an initial decision must often be made as to which is the dominant problem, in order to treat that one first. Sometimes more than one therapy can be used at the same time (such as bladder training for the unstable bladder, combined with pelvic floor exercises for stress incontinence). Other combinations of problems should be treated one at a time: for example, an unstable bladder and outflow obstruction. The instability, if dominant, should be treated first, because if outflow resistance is lowered the incontinence is likely to worsen.

These mixed pathologies should always be considered when assessing the incontinent elderly.

Hormone changes

The urethra and trigone in the female are formed embryologically from the same hormone-dependent tissue as the vagina. When fully oestrogenised, the surface of the urethral wall is very soft and convoluted, forming many folds which interdigitate to form an efficient water-tight seal (Figure 8.1).

(a) Side view   (b) Cross-section

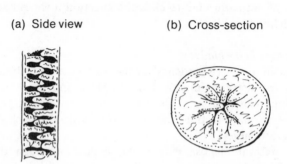

Figure 8.1 *Well-oestrogenised urethra (note interdigitating folds giving efficient closure).*

Oestrogen levels do not usually drop for ten years after the menopause, and many women maintain a good oestrogenisation well into old age. However, if hormone levels do fall the walls of the urethra become a lot less soft and the folds less pronounced, so that closure is less efficient (Figure 8.2). Coupled with decreased mucus production, which lowers surface tension, the result is that both stress incontinence and leakage during uninhibited detrusor contractions are more likely to arise.

(a) Side view   (b) Cross-section

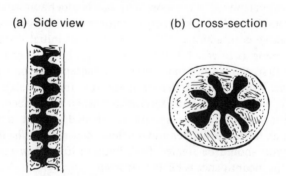

Figure 8.2 *Oestrogen-deficient urethra.*

With increasing age a larger area of the urethra and trigone become oestrogen-sensitive. Lack of oestrogen may cause a urethritis and trigonitis. The patient will suffer symptoms similar to cystitis – dysuria, frequency and often urgency. This will be associated with a vaginitis ('atrophic' or 'senile' vaginitis), which can be detected easily by looking at the vulva which will appear red, inflamed, and often dry. There may be secondary infection. Much of the perineal discomfort commonly attributed to urine and incontinence in elderly women is probably in fact a symptom of atrophic vaginitis. Considerable excoriation, and even adhesions, may develop. If the diagnosis is in doubt a histological smear will confirm it.

Oestrogen replacement therapy will remedy these conditions. Ideally this should be a very low dose (0.1mcg per day). Unfortunately, no commercial preparation is yet available in such a dose and the nearest is a stilboestrol pessary 0.5mcg, which can be given vaginally on alternate nights. Oestrogen is also available as a cream (e.g. dienoestrol cream), but many old people find the vaginal applicators difficult or uncomfortable to use, and doses tend to be loaded into the applicators inaccurately. Oral preparations (e.g. Premarin tablets) are available for those who cannot manage a vaginal dose. (Considerable dexterity is necessary for vaginal application and some women find it distasteful or impossible, particularly the nulliparous.) Oral oestrogens may carry a higher risk of side-effects. Oestrogens should not be used for women with a history of thrombo-embolic disease or malignancy of the reproductive system. On a low dose the therapy can be given continuously or via a '3-month on, 3-month off' basis. Withdrawal bleeding is rare. Patients should be warned that with pessaries or cream used at night they may get a white discharge on rising in the morning. They should be advised that this is of no importance as the active hormone will have already been absorbed.

The prostate

Prostatic hypertrophy is dealt with elsewhere (Chapter 7). The incidence of prostatic malignancy increases greatly in old age and is present in 30% of men over seventy, rising to 80% over ninety. Most of these malignancies are latent and do not affect life expectancy. However, the possibility of an active tumour should be borne in mind with men who experience an altered micturition pattern, especially difficulty in passing urine. Age is no bar to surgery and a transurethral resection is a relatively quick and safe solution to prostatic hypertrophy, whether benign or malignant.

There has been considerable controversy in recent years over whether a female equivalent of the prostate exists. It has been suggested that this 'female prostatic homologue' (possibly the para-urethral glands) may explain some voiding difficulties in elderly women. However there has, as yet, been no clear evidence of hypertrophy causing bladder-neck obstruction.

Neurological deterioration

Ageing and neurological disease make all the varieties of neurological bladder dysfunction more common in old age. Predominant is detrusor instability, with a very high proportion of all old people having some degree of instability. Among the incontinent elderly it is the most common bladder problem.

Neurogenic voiding difficulties can occur in all the complex combinations described in Chapter 10. It is also likely that with the increased incidence of autonomic neuropathy associated with ageing, the number of both men and women with functional (non-anatomic) obstruction from detrusor-sphincter dyssynergia increases. The urethral sphincters do not relax completely during micturition and a degree of residual urine, possibly with overflow incontinence, develops.

Bladder sensation often changes with age. Instead of appreciating the sensation of bladder filling at about half of capacity, as younger people do, many of the elderly first feel the desire to void at, or very near, bladder capacity. To the active and mobile old person this can represent a considerable inconvenience, as they will have to stop whatever they are doing and find a lavatory. To the immobile elderly, or to someone with an unstable bladder or painful arthritis, this will often result in incontinence: there simply is not enough time between sensation and unavoidable micturition to prevent incontinence.

Mental impairment

Most people become mentally less flexible and adaptable to some extent as they age. Many react with confusion and even aggression to circumstances which have suddenly or unexpectedly altered. Some suffer accelerated age changes, resulting in dementia. The specific problems and management of the mentally impaired elderly incontinent person are dealt with later in this chapter.

Diabetes

Over the age of seventy, 30% of women and 20% of men have diabetes. However mild a form of the disease is present, it can have a profound effect upon the bladder, particularly causing atony (see Chapter 10).

Many of the atonic bladders seen in old age are directly related to diabetic neuropathy.

Undiagnosed diabetes may present as polyuria and polydipsia; vulval irritation with reddened swollen labia and possibly a candida albicans infection; or with an atonic bladder with overflow incontinnence. Screening for diabetes should be routine among the elderly with urinary symptoms. If a urine test detects sugar, a glucose tolerance test is usually then performed to confirm the diagnosis.

The influence of other disorders

Multiple pathology is common in old age. Many elderly people with bladder or bowel problems also have other disorders to contend with, many of which will affect the ability to be continent. Neurological disorders not only directly influence bladder function but also often impair ability to cope with it. A Parkinsonian tremor or a hemiparesis may make independent toileting slow, or even impossible. Heart or lung disease may make the patient so slow or breathless that the lavatory cannot be reached in time. Arthritis may limit mobility and dexterity. Depression is common in old age and may lead to apathy, self-neglect and incontinence. Alcoholism may likewise be overlooked as a reason for gradual deterioration in mental and physical state, with concomitant incontinence. Treatment of these disorders may result in a consequent improvement in continence.

Drugs

Just as many other disorders may be present, multiple drug regimes are also common. So many drugs have side-effects on bladder function that this is often a contributory factor in causing incontinence (see Table 2.2). Rationalisation of a drug regime, excluding unnecessary prescription, will often improve, if not cure, the problem. This may be lowering the dose of diuretics, or using a less rapidly acting one; decreasing sedation; or switching to an alternative medication for a particular disorder (e.g. amitriptyline to dothiepin where the former is causing voiding difficulties for the depressed patient).

Fluids and the elderly

The habit of restricting fluids to control incontinence can reach dangerous proportions in some old people, who may drink almost nothing. Many already have a precarious metabolic stability, and severe fluid and electrolyte imbalance may result. Dehydration, malaise, constipation and confusion can follow.

Older people often find drinking large quantities of fluid difficult, as it makes them feel bloated. When encouraging the elderly to drink reasonably (ideally more than one litre per twenty-four hours), it is important to find out what they like and when they prefer to drink. Many who find water or squash unpalatable can drink the same volume of strong tea or stout with little problem (providing, of course, that the preferred drink does not aggravate the bladder).

ATTITUDES AND THE IMPORTANCE OF THE ENVIRONMENT

An environment in which the attitudes of those around the old person – whether relatives, friends, or care staff – are such that each individual is expected to be continent, often achieves the desired effect. Where it is taken for granted that, past a certain age or with certain diseases or disabilities, incontinence is inevitable, the old person often lacks both the incentive and the opportunity to be continent. Where everything possible is done to prevent incontinence and to treat it when it does occur, the likelihood of continence is much higher.

Promotion of continence among the elderly involves creating an environment in which they can easily and safely cope with bladder and bowel function, whether or not this function is disordered.

Independence

The greater the independence that the environment allows, the greater is the older person's potential for continence, both because of the need for privacy and the increased urgency that many of them experience. Many are reticent in asking for help and there may not always be someone immediately available when needed.

Beds should be at the correct height for the individual to be able to get out of easily (adjustable-height beds are ideal in hospital). The bed should not be too soft or sag in the middle, as this can make rising difficult. Chairs should also be of the correct height, not too soft or deep, and have armrests at an appropriate height to aid leverage.

A good walking-aid, whether stick, tripod, or frame, can greatly improve mobility, speed, and confidence in visiting the lavatory independently.

Clothes should be easy to adjust and any incontinence aid should, where possible, be capable of easy removal and replacement by the user.

The lavatory
Lavatories should have a door which is easy to open and lock. The seat must be the correct height for easy sitting and rising. (See Chapter 9 for modifications which can be made, and alternative urinals and commodes for those who cannot get to the lavatory.)

Distance
An old person generally needs to be much nearer to a lavatory than a younger person in order to be reliably continent. Because many feel sensation only at or near capacity, urgency is often considerable. Once urgency is felt it may not be possible for the old person to rush. The Scottish Home and Health Department have estimated that 30–40 feet is the optimum distance between the elderly person's starting point and the lavatory. This means situating lavatories near day areas in homes, hospitals and day centres, and may involve structural alterations in the patient's own home. The route also needs to be unobstructed and without stairs if mobility is limited.

Signposting
In unfamiliar surroundings, being able to identify the correct lavatory quickly and easily is important. Clear signposts in public places (including hospital wards) and clear labels on doors are important. It is easy to understand that someone who has misinterpreted a 'ladies' or 'gents' symbol (and some, such as Edwardian hats and bonnets, can easily be mistaken by anyone) may be unwilling to go out for fear that the same will happen again. Colour-coded lavatory doors and unambiguous well-lit signs at an appropriate height are a great help to the elderly.

EMOTIONAL AND PSYCHOLOGICAL FACTORS

As with younger patients, psychological factors are important with the elderly, although a direct causative role is unproven. Incontinence may be observed to start following bereavement or some other stressful event (notably admission to residential care) in some patients. Occasionally, incontinence may be seen as deliberate, conscious attention-seeking behaviour. This cannot simply be dismissed as of no consequence. If someone feels the need to gain the attention of other human beings in this drastic manner, it should surely alert professionals to the fact that the individual is fairly desperate and is receiving insufficient attention for his more positive attributes in life. If a manipulative person discovers he can gain the attention he craves by being incontinent, he is likely to repeat the behaviour. An individual assessment might indicate more productive channels for this desired human contact.

TREATMENT OF INCONTINENCE IN THE ELDERLY

The incontinent old person should have incontinence investigated and treated as anyone else would. A good nursing assessment (see Chapter 3) will reveal many problems which can be remedied, but for those who do not respond to nursing measures a full urodynamic assessment is usually desirable. Few old people find this unduly distressing or uncomfortable if conducted in a private and relaxed atmosphere.

The full range of treatments are applicable to the elderly incontinent. As with younger people, the options should be explained and the decision made jointly with the patient. Some old people are reluctant to undergo invasive treatment such as surgery, and prefer reliable containment. Drug therapy should be used with care in the elderly, as many are more sensitive to side-effects than younger people, but provided they are introduced cautiously and gradually, all the standard preparations may be used. Time spent teaching the patient should increase his understanding and compliance with prescribed regimes. With improvements in surgical techniques and safer anaesthetics, surgery is increasingly feasible for those older people who need it.

The special problems of the elderly resident in institutions are dealt with in Chapter 11.

INTERMITTENT CATHETERISATION

(A fuller discussion of the techniques involved is given in Chapter 10.)

Voiding problems and large volumes of post-micturition residual urine become increasingly common with advancing age. Where surgical or pharmacological treatments are inappropriate or unsuccessful, the use of intermittent catheterisation should be considered. Many elderly people retain sufficient dexterity to catheterise themselves, although the urethral meatus may be more difficult to find if it migrates along the vaginal wall. If the patient cannot manage, a spouse or relative may learn the procedure. Otherwise nursing help must be employed. Whether in hospital or community, if removing the residual urine will keep the patient continent, every effort should be made to ensure that this is done. Older people often require intermittent catheterisation far less frequently than younger people with voiding problems (see Chapter 10), as often the residual urine accumulates gradually. Once per day, or even on alternate days, is sometimes enough to restore continence. With a proportion of patients bladder function will return over a period of weeks, so that catheterisation can be discontinued as residual volumes drop.

Instituting an intermittent catheterisation regime, on a ward or in the community, often involves a considerable readjustment of nursing routines (and attitudes). Once the idea has been accepted and the appropriate equipment ordered (such as adequate numbers of catheter packs and a good angle-poise light), it soon becomes routine. Nurses become acquainted with any anatomical idiosyncrasies of the patient and each catheterisation only takes a few minutes, especially if timing is planned to fit in with the individual patient's daily routine (e.g. before getting up in the morning, so that he does not have to get undressed and dressed again). It must be emphasised that when a nurse performs a catheterisation this should always be done aseptically, because of the risks of cross-infection. If the patient or a relative is doing it at home a clean technique is perfectly acceptable (see Ch. 10).

INCONTINENCE IN TERMINAL ILLNESS

Many people become incontinent, often doubly, in the final stages of a terminal illness. This can be a tremendous burden on carers and a humiliation for the sufferer, if he is aware of what is happening. Incontinence of urine may be because of any of the causes outlined elsewhere in this book. Most likely are neurological disease, cerebral clouding, often exacerbated by immobility and loss of independence. Faecal incontinence can often be prevented by good bowel management – to prevent constipation and impaction or to regulate the neurogenic bowel (see Chapter 14).

Obviously vigorous investigation will seldom be desirable for the terminally ill person, but even so some incontinence can be cured by sensible prescription of drugs for detrusor instability, the use of hand-held urinals for the immobile, and by alerting carers to the need for regular toileting. If incontinence persists, a good aid or appliance may well control it. If leakage is heavy or movement to a urinal or commode becomes painful and difficult, an indwelling catheter should be seen as a positive alternative. Long-term risks can be discounted, and a catheter may enable the dying person to spend his last days at home. Relatives can sleep or go out without worrying that the patient may need to micturate or will be lying in a puddle.

A bladder or bowel fistula as part of a terminal illness can prove tremendously distressing, and is one of the most difficult problems to deal with. Probably the most effective management is to use large high-quality body-worn pads (e.g. Mölnlycke Tenaform Super), or a diaper-style garment (e.g. Peaudouce Slipad). Scrupulous skin care and hygiene are essential.

Uncontrolled incontinence certainly makes the development of a pressure sore more likely, and in an emaciated person this risk is increased. For women, a catheter should prevent this occurring and thereby avoid extra pain and distress. Men may find a penile sheath is as effective as a catheter.

THE ELDERLY MENTALLY INFIRM

The majority of elderly people do not become mentally infirm. For those who do, there is a great spectrum of impairment, from slight memory loss and coarsening of personality traits to severe confusion and dementia. If impairment is severe, the individual may need institutional care. However, the majority of elderly mentally infirm are cared for by relatives in their own homes.

Incontinence is seldom an inevitable feature of memory loss or dementia. Many demented people are not incontinent, and continence is so deeply ingrained in most people that it is often one of the last social skills to be lost. Too often other causes of incontinence are overlooked and left untreated. The individual may be faecally impacted, have a urinary tract infection, or be immobile (King, 1979; 1980). Any of the bladder dysfunctions may be present. A concomitant illness such as diabetes or depression may be the real cause of incontinence. Indeed, in the elderly, depression may mimic dementia.

The elderly mentally infirm are even more dependent than the fit elderly on their surroundings for their level of functioning. Many of those living in their own homes, with familiar people and objects, can maintain a relatively normal lifestyle, even with quite advanced mental impairment. Sometimes incontinence results from disorientation, especially in changed surroundings. It is very difficult for demented people to learn new things, and they may never become accustomed to a strange environment, even after prolonged residence. In a hospital or a home, good signposting and lighting coupled with appropriate reminders may help. However, as already discussed, many old people retain Victorian attitudes to elimination, and may well deny their need for the lavatory if not asked discreetly. A nurse asking publicly and in a loud voice will often be met with a refusal or denial, even hostility.

It is important to expect continence. Too often the demented are simply expected to be incontinent and not given the opportunity or encouragement to be dry. In institutions, the routine may be geared to everyone being incontinent, with regular washing and changing routines. Indeed, it can be easier for staff, in the short term, to have a monotonous regular routine rather than struggle to rehabilitate or retrain (Wells, 1975).

A behavioural assessment of each individual will give much information as to why incontinence might be occurring. Many 'psychogeriatric' units have a clinical psychologist attached, and in some places a community psychologist or community psychiatric nurse specialising in the care of the elderly is available. These people can often be helpful in contributing to the assessment. If the incontinent individual is unable to communicate his needs verbally, he should be closely observed for any typical behaviour occurring prior to micturition, e.g. getting up, wandering, pulling at clothing, other verbal or non-verbal cues. If such cues are discovered and all carers made aware of them, needs can be responded to appropriately. By discovering the patient's past and present life history (what sort of person he was, what were his interests, activities, pet hates), it may be possible to deduce that incontinence is a symptom of apathy, protest or despair at a currently unacceptable life situation. If someone who has always been a solitary and shy person is expected to become accustomed to living, sleeping, dressing, and eating with twenty-five other people whom he neither knows nor likes, it is not difficult to see why a formerly fastidious personality might crumble under the strain. Many people do become incontinent on admission to residential care (whether a home or hospital), or soon after, and this may be related to the loss of independence, personal responsibility, and sense of self-worth that often accompanies such admission. It may also happen when being obliged to sell a home and move in with children.

Some people seem to employ the defence mechanism of regression under such circumstances – becoming passive, dependent and often incontinent. By regressing to an infantile state they may be able to avoid facing the reality of their unacceptable situation. Occasionally incontinence can be interpreted as an expression of anger, as one of the few weapons available to the individual to use against his carers. It may be noted that incontinence occurs only when one particular carer is around. It may occur with certain disliked activities or events (e.g. while being dressed or when 'pop' music is on the radio) but not with preferred activities (e.g. during occupational therapy or watching certain TV programmes). It is often observed that patients who are seemingly 'hopelessly' incontinent on a ward may be dry for a whole day on a coach trip.

What happens after incontinence occurs is also important. In some circumstances incontinence may become rewarding, since it gains attention and creates a fuss. This is especially true in a socially impoverished situation such as an understaffed institution. The individual may get very little attention when dry or going to the lavatory independently – the staff are busy giving care to those who really need it. If incontinent, however, the individual will usually gain attention, often promptly. A member of staff will come, talk, touch, and usually smile. He may be taken to the bathroom for a wash or to be changed. Even if the staff member is angry or hostile this may be better than no communication at all. The continent person may have nobody talk to him between breakfast and lunch. The incontinent person gains physical and social contact every time incontinence occurs. Great care must be taken not to attribute incontinence automatically to deliberate attention-seeking. It is seldom a conscious choice, especially for the confused person. However, it is important to be alert to staff practices which unwittingly reinforce the very behaviour that is least wanted. The same may be true of patients in the community. The incontinent person may benefit from considerably increased attention (e.g. the supplies man delivering pads, the home help to wash the sheets, the bath nurse, may all start to visit) whereas before becoming incontinent very few people visited. Again, it should not be interpreted as the patient's conscious choice to remain incontinent, but there is certainly little incentive to try to remain dry.

In advanced dementia all social realisation of the desirability of continence may be lost. The individual may become completely uninhibited and, with no reason to try to hang on, will pass urine and faeces as and when he needs to. If the concept of a right and wrong place becomes meaningless, then clothes, bed, floor, or furniture may be used indiscriminately. Urine and faeces are no longer seen as dirty or unpleasant, and may be played with or smeared when discovered. This will often seem particularly unacceptable behaviour to relatives or staff. Sometimes the recognition of what a lavatory is meant for is lost, so that even when taken to one, it is not used appropriately. The patient may sit and do nothing, then be incontinent soon afterwards, or the restless person may refuse to sit at all. Alternatively, the distinction between a lavatory and other receptacles is lost, so that urine or faeces are passed into wastepaper bins, buckets, or any other receptacle which is to hand.

Most people have a lifetime's conditioned reflex to pass urine while seated with no clothing over the genital area, on a lavatory in privacy and with the sensation of a full bladder. The demented are very dependent upon familiar stimuli in order to maintain their activities. It is all too easy to upset these conditioned reflexes by offering confusing stimuli (Newman, 1962). The individual may be repeatedly taken to the lavatory when the bladder is not full, if no one has found out the most likely times he will need to go. Often demented people who are being looked after lead very regular lives – with meals and drinks served at routine times every day. Each person's bladder will react differently to this – no two people are likely to have an identical pattern of micturition, but the pattern for each individual is likely to be similar each day. An accurate chart will reveal any such pattern. If a confused person is repeatedly taken to the lavatory and does not need to use it, his concept of the purpose of the lavatory will be destroyed. Likewise, a lack of privacy may militate against his use of the lavatory. At other times the person may be sat, with no underwear on ('What is the point if he is incontinent?') in a chair in a quiet corner, and need to pass urine. Sitting with a bare bottom on an underpad on the chair, the obvious message seems to be: 'Go ahead – pass urine here'. This can lead to paradoxical urination patterns – the individual does not pass urine if taken to the lavatory but is incontinent as soon as he is relaxed, quiet, and comfortable again in a chair or bed. This can be most frustrating and annoying for the carers, who often feel the behaviour is deliberate. It must be understood that the individual is seldom trying to be awkward but is merely responding to the confusing mixed stimuli to which he is subjected.

It is common for demented people to deny their incontinence. Sometimes they are well aware of the problem but are too ashamed to admit it to others. This can lead to attempting to hide the evidence – concealing soiled clothes or pads in a cupboard, putting a clean sheet over a soiled one. Often the situation can become most unpleasant before anyone realises what is happening. If confronted, the person may become hostile and abusive or try to blame someone else (or the cat). Sometimes the person may be denying the situation even to himself, and be so distressed by his incontinence that he genuinely does not consciously know that it is happening. Often in advanced dementia the individual will be as oblivious of incontinence as he seems to be of his surroundings.

Reality orientation

It is very important to maintain a reality-orientated environment for the confused elderly, in order to keep as many conditioned responses to normal cues operative as possible. It has often been noted in hospitals that if patients are dressed in their own clothes (including appropriate underwear), and have their own possessions around them with plenty of stimulation and activities, incontinence is much less frequent. Information must be repeated frequently if it is to be retained. Staff should use the patient's own name often, in the form which the patient prefers (whether first name or surname or a lifelong nickname). Frequent use of diminutive endearments ('dearie', 'love') do little to keep the individual in touch. Conversation should include repeated use of reality cues – about time, place, weather, family or events. Clear, easily-read clocks, calendars and signposts at an appropriate height can all help failing memories. Most institutions are attempting to move away from the large, featureless day area where everyone sits around on plastic chairs in a large circle (making any eye contact or communication difficult), with the endless drone of a TV set no one is watching. Even within the constraints of staff and resource shortages, many small alterations can be made towards individualising care. Covering a hospital locker with photos and reminders of family, friends and former home, or having a large mirror with the person's name clearly written above his reflection, may help to remind the patient who he is. While recent memory may be poor, longer-term memories may be intact, and old records, picture books or conversations about the war (usually the first world war) often bring pleasure and recognition. People who are seemingly very confused may still be able to perform a lifetime's repetitive activity – a housewife may help with bedmaking, even if the result is slow and somewhat untidy. Art, drama and occupational therapy should all be used to the full where available. Many long-stay units now have pets (such as a cat or budgie), outings, and frequent voluntary visitors. By keeping people as stimulated and occupied and as motivated as possible, and by using carefully planned repeated information for teaching, it is possible to maximise the level of functioning of confused people. This is of course desirable in its own right. As an added bonus continence is often greatly improved.

Behaviour modification

Behaviour modification techniques may be used to help the confused elderly to be continent, in much the same way as for the mentally handicapped (see Chapter 12). By reinforcing the desired behaviour (i.e. continence, and passing urine in the correct place) and extinguishing the undesired behaviour (i.e. incontinence), it is often possible to use the theories of operant conditioning to promote continence.

The aim is to reverse the attention pattern outlined above – to give attention, praise and physical contact for continence, and withdraw these when incontinence occurs. To be effective, everyone who comes into contact with the patient must understand and carry out the procedure, so that consistency is maintained. Every time someone approaches the individual and he is dry, he should be rewarded (by a smile, praise, a hug – an appropriate reinforcer should be chosen for each patient). If using the lavatory correctly, or indicating the need to go appropriately, the reinforcement should be given as promptly as possible. When incontinence occurs it must, of course, be dealt with, but this should be done with a minimal amount of fuss and attention – no smiles, no conversation, and minimal physical contact. Punishment is not warranted. This procedure can be used for day incontinence (Grosicki, 1968), or night incontinence (Hartie and Black, 1975; Barker, 1979), and will, if used consistently over a sufficiently long period (often several months), restore continence for some individuals. It is often possible to teach relatives to use such a programme at home if they are highly motivated.

Advanced dementia

In the advanced stages of dementia all these attempts to achieve continence might fail. It is important that carers (whether relatives or staff) are not made to feel guilty or inadequate because of such failures. For some people incontinence does become inevitable, even with the best available care and treatment. At present we have to accept this. Regular toileting, if the individual will use the toilet, may 'catch' some of the incontinence in the daytime, especially if it is timed to coincide with the most likely times as revealed by an incontinence chart. There seems little point in repeated awakenings at night – the patient will often become more confused if tired, and will usually benefit more from a good night's sleep than from repeated toileting, unless obviously awake and agitated.

Probably the most important aspect of care is to provide high-quality incontinence pads, in ample quantities, and of a type which are as easy as possible to use. A good pad will protect the skin, protect the environment and clothing, minimise odour, and maintain the dignity of the individual. (The selection and use of incontinence aids is discussed in detail in Chapter 13.) Wherever the demented person is being cared for, it should be possible to relieve many of the most unacceptable aspects of his incontinence, and allow him to spend his last years in relative comfort.

REFERENCES AND FURTHER READING

Barker, P., 1979. 'Nocturnal enuresis; an experimental study involving two behavioural approaches'. *International Journal of Nursing Studies*, 16, 319–327.

Brocklehurst, J. C., Dillane, J. B., Griffiths, L., Fry, J., 1968. 'The prevalence and symptomatology of urinary infection in an aged population'. *Gerontologica Clinica*, 10, 242–253.

Brocklehurst, J. C., 1977. 'The causes and management of incontinence in the elderly'. *Nursing Mirror*, 144, 15.

Brocklehurst, J. C., 1978. 'The genitourinary system'. In: Brocklehurst, J. C. (ed.), *Textbook of Geriatic Medicine and Gerontology* (2nd edn.). Churchill Livingstone, Edinburgh and London.

Browne, B., 1978. *Management for Continence*. Age Concern (England), Mitcham, Surrey.

Clay, E. C., 1978. 'Incontinence of urine'. *Nursing Mirror*, 146, 10, 36–38; 146, 11, 23–24.

Grosicki, J. P., 1968. 'Effect of operant conditioning on modification of incontinence in neuropsychiatric geriatric patients'. *Nursing Research*, 17, 304–311.

Hartie, A., Black, D., 1975. 'A dry bed is the objective'. *Nursing Times*, 71, 1874–1876.

Irvine, R., 1983. 'Continence in the elderly'. *Nursing Times*, 79, 17, 45–48.

King, M. R., 1979. 'A study of incontinence in a psychiatric hospital'. *Nursing Times*, 75, 26, 1133–1135.

King, M. R., 1980. 'Treatment of incontinence'. *Nursing Times*, 76, 23, 1006–1010.

Lepine, A., Renault, R. K., Stewart, I. D., 1979. 'The incidence and management of incontinence in a home for the elderly'. *Health and Social Service Journal*, 89, 4639, E9–E12.

Millard, P. H., 1979. 'The promotion of continence'. *Health Trends*, 11, 27–28.

Newman, J. L., 1962. 'Old folks in wet beds'. *British Medical Journal*, 1, 1824–1827.

Sanford, J. R., 1975. 'Tolerance of debility in elderly dependants by supporters at home: its significance for hospital practice'. *British Medical Journal*, 3, 471–473.

Schwartz, D. R., 1977. 'Personal point of view – a report of 17 elderly patients with a persistent problem of urinary incontinence'. *Health Bulletin*, 35, 4, 197–204.

Volpe, A., Kastenbaum, R., 1967. 'Beer and TLC'. *American Journal of Nursing*, 67, 100–103.

Wells, T., 1975. 'Promoting urinary continence in the elderly in hospital'. *Nursing Times*, 71, 48, 1908–1909.

Willington, F. L., 1975. *Incontinence.* Nursing Times publication, Macmillan, London.

Willington, F. L. (ed.), 1976. *Incontinence in the elderly.* Academic Press, London.

Chapter 9

Aids to Continence for the Physically Disabled

Many physically disabled people have a neurogenic bladder problem which impairs their continence. Chapter 10 discusses the different types of neurogenic bladder and their management. However, many disabled people are rendered incontinent not by a bladder problem, but by a poorly adapted environment. Even those with completely normal bladder function may become incontinent if physical difficulties are severe enough. This chapter considers methods by which the physically handicapped may be helped to be independently continent. The aids to toileting mentioned in this chapter, together with many more, are listed in the Association of Continence Advisors' (this spelling) *Directory of Aids to Toileting* (1985). This directory gives details of suppliers, approximate price and dimensions of items available in the UK.

CONTINENCE IN PUBLIC PLACES

Many public buildings and amenities are poorly equipped for the needs of disabled people, especially regarding the provision of suitable lavatories. Although toilets for the disabled are becoming more common, especially in new buildings, there are still many situations in which it is impossible for someone with limited mobility to reach a lavatory. Many obstacles are obvious, such as a flight of steps, a door too narrow to admit a walking aid or wheelchair, or an inwardly opening door in a cubicle too small to allow the door to be closed with a wheelchair inside. Other obstacles are more subtle, such as poor signposting or ambiguous labels on doors which handicap the partially sighted. Where there are no facilities specifically designed for the disabled, wheelchair access is seldom possible, and an escort of the opposite sex cannot accompany and help. Lavatories on trains and planes are notably small and awkward.

All too often the disabled person is excluded from activities, not because of his physical disabilities, but because the lavatory facilities are inadequate. Journeys or holidays are difficult unless facilities are already known to the individual. Shopping must always be done in centres with a 'disabled' lavatory. Visits to the cinema, theatre, or other places of entertainment must always be preceded by enquiries. Going to a pub for a drink is often impossible. Some even have to give up a job which they are perfectly capable of doing because the nearest lavatory is two floors down. Even where there are specially designed facilities, access to them is not always guaranteed. Some are poorly designed, without reference to available guidelines, and may just have a grab-rail as a token gesture. Sometimes a tried and trusted convenience is suddenly closed because of vandalism, lack of staff, or as part of expenditure cut-backs. Time and time again the activities of the physically disabled are determined not by personal preference but by public provision for their needs.

This situation is improving, and public awareness increasing. Most new public buildings now have reasonable facilities. Even those not covered by legislation, such as private hotels, often have specially constructed rooms for the disabled. Some districts have entered a scheme of keeping toilets for the disabled locked (National Key Scheme), and issuing all registered disabled people with a key, to avoid vandalism. The Royal Association for Disability and Rehabilitation (RADAR) publish a guide to accessible public lavatories, giving details of location, parking, access, and opening hours (RADAR, 1984).

LAVATORY DESIGN FOR THE DISABLED

Public conveniences
The British Standards Institution (1979) issues a *Code of Practice for Access for the Disabled to Buildings*, which makes detailed recommendations on lavatory design for both ambulant and wheelchair-bound disabled people. Figure 9.1 (overleaf) shows a cubicle layout to accommodate a wheelchair. The door should open outwards or slide, unless the room is large, because an inward-opening door takes up too much space. Handles, locks and rails should be large enough to grasp easily, simple to use with minimal strength, and low enough to reach easily from a wheelchair.

A cubicle of at least 1.5m x 2m should allow transfer from a wheelchair either from in front or from the side. Some people can

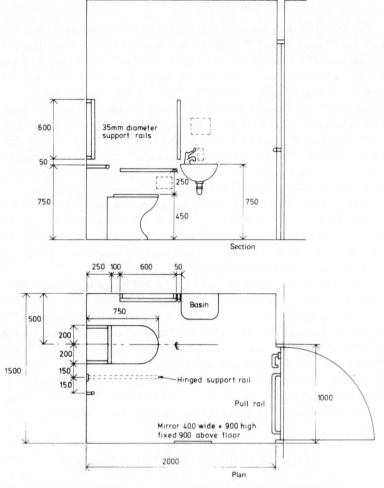

Figure 9.1 *Lavatory design allowing wheelchair access (British Standards Institution BS 5810: 1979, by permission). Dimensions in millimetres. Positions for paper holder, soap dispenser and towel dispenser are shown dotted. A disposal bin should be provided.*

stand and turn with the chair in front of the lavatory; others prefer to remove one arm from the wheelchair and transfer sideways. A few use a chair with a zipped back so that they can transfer backwards (this is particularly appropriate for double amputees).

The BSI recommends at least one unisex facility in a range of public amenities: e.g. shopping centres, large department stores, transport, health, recreation and entertainment buildings.

Private lavatories

The lavatory in the disabled person's own home can be tailored to his particular needs. There may of course be limitations because of the needs of other members of the household.

In certain cases a home improvement grant may be obtained from the local council to build a completely new bathroom, for example downstairs for someone who can no longer manage to get upstairs. This is not always feasible if space is limited. The local housing department should be consulted for advice on what is available and how to apply.

There is a wide variety of toilet frames and grab rails. These can add greatly to the stability and confidence of someone unsteady on his feet, and give leverage for rising from a wheelchair or the lavatory. Some are free-standing. For long-term use it is generally preferable to have rails fixed either to the floor or to the walls. Flanges at the feet of a frame give added stability. Horizontal, vertical or diagonal variations are available, depending on the individual's needs. The Disabled Living Foundation's notes on Personal Care (List 7B) gives details.

The lavatory seat should be at a height that is easy to get on and off. People with stiff or painful joints may find it difficult to use a modern low-level lavatory. A footstool may be needed to give the correct sitting position on a high seat. People transferring sideways from a wheelchair to the lavatory must have each seat at the same height as the other. Detachable raised lavatory seats can be used to increase the height from between two and seven inches. It is important to use a model with an inner lip fitting directly into the bowl (not perched on top of the ordinary seat), as these are the most stable. Some raised seats have a cut-out front to facilitate wiping. Adjustable clips will ensure stability. Others slope forward or sideways to accommodate a rigid leg or caliper. The seat should be easily removed for cleaning as well as for when the lavatory is used by others.

Spring-loaded or electrically operated elevating lavatory seats can be obtained if rising is a particular problem, although they should be used with care for a frail person, who might be catapulted forward. Padded or inflatable seats may be more comfortable for those who take a particularly long time to empty the bowel or bladder, or for those at risk of developing pressure sores. Wooden seats tend to be more comfortable than plastic, and a bench seat will allow sliding.

Toilet paper should be situated within easy reach, without the user having to stretch. For those with the use of only one hand, the paper must be situated on the side they can use. A roll of paper is very difficult to tear off with one hand, and people may be tempted to try dangerous manoeuvres such as holding the roll still with the forehead. Folded paper in a pull-out dispenser is much easier for the one-handed. People who have a problem with wiping because of limited reach may find toilet tongs or a bottom wiper (Nottingham Aids) useful. These hold the toilet paper and extend the reach considerably. Alternatively, a portable bidet (Ganmill) which fits on top of the lavatory pan can be used. This will usually require the presence of a helper as the bidet has to be filled with warm water, positioned on the pan, and emptied after use via a plug into the lavatory. Where finances and space permit, a permanent bidet with foot controls (e.g. Clos-o-Mat) may be useful.

ALTERNATIVES TO THE LAVATORY

If the individual cannot get onto a lavatory, the use of an alternative receptacle can enable continence to be maintained. The selection of an alternative will depend on the user's needs and preferences.

Commodes

There are many different commodes available, from a simple stool to very sophisticated designs. It is important to make sure that a commode is the correct height and acceptable to the user and family. Some people dislike the idea of a commode in living areas or the bedroom, especially if others are around. This is often forgotten on hospital wards, where patients may be expected to use a bedside commode at night without curtains to screen the user from the view of other patients. However, for many people a commode is a real benefit, especially if mobility is slow or painful, or nocturia very frequent. Some commodes are wooden rather than metal and can be disguised as an easy-chair. Optional features include removable arms (for sideways transfer from a wheelchair or bed), wheels, and footrests. Some are foldable so that they can easily be taken away on holiday. Some can be wheeled over a lavatory and so used as a sanitary chair with the pan removed. Others can be fixed to the side of the bed for stability in night use. When assessing the individual for choice of commode, his height and weight should be taken into account. Generally, a commode will be between 475mm and 550mm high, although many are adjustable. Special commodes are available for the very obese, with splayed legs for added stability.

A commode must be fitted with a compatible container, which fits the aperture closely, to avoid soiling of the commode or floor. Usually, it is most convenient to be able to remove the pan from the back. The Institute of Consumer Ergonomics, Loughborough, has also recommended that commodes have a cover which is light and hinged at the back; padded arms, which are level and extend forward as far as the front of the seat; a seat and arms made from non-absorbent material; and a container which is easy to remove, carry and replace.

The Disabled Living Foundation's List 7A (Personal Toilet) gives details and suppliers of the variations available.

Chemical toilets

Chemical toilets, designed for use in camping or caravanning, may be used instead of a commode, for instance in situations where the user is unable to empty a commode and has no regular helper. The chemicals ensure that even if it is not emptied for several days, urine and faeces do not cause a smell or infection risk.

When either a commode or chemical toilet has to be used in a living-room it may be possible to partition off a corner of the room with a ceiling-to-floor curtain, so that some privacy and separation is maintained.

Male hand-held urinals (Figure 9.2, overleaf)

Ideally a hand-held urinal should be easy to use independently, easy to empty and clean or to dispose of, and spill-proof. The standard male 'bottle' or urinal is familiar to most nurses (Figure 9.2(a)). It is available in metal, glass, plastic or disposable papier-maché, the latter two being lighter for those with a weak grip. Bottles have a capacity of 500ml or 1 litre. Some have a snap-close lid to avoid the danger of spilling after use. A bedside or chairside holder is useful to prevent a full bottle being accidentally kicked or knocked over. A flatter version may be more stable to use and less easy to spill if placed between the legs in bed (Figure 9.2(b)). A non-spill adapter will fit most standard bottles (Figure 9.2(c)). The rubber sleeve fits snugly into the neck of the bottle with the air vent upwards. The valve allows urine to pass in but not to return. This is particularly useful for someone with a poor grip or shaky hands who tends to spill or drop the bottle, or someone who falls asleep with a used bottle in bed and then rolls over and knocks it over.

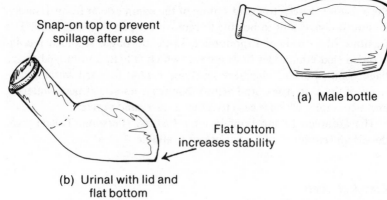

Snap-on top to prevent
spillage after use

(a) Male bottle

Flat bottom
increases stability

(b) Urinal with lid and
flat bottom

Figure 9.2
Male hand-held urinals.

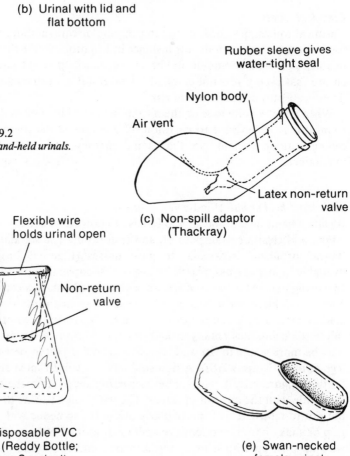

Rubber sleeve gives
water-tight seal

Nylon body

Air vent

Latex non-return
valve

(c) Non-spill adaptor
(Thackray)

Flexible wire
holds urinal open

Non-return
valve

(d) Disposable PVC
urinal (Reddy Bottle;
Downs Surgical)

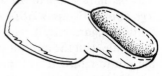

(e) Swan-necked
female urinal

The Reddy Bottle (Figure 9.2(d)) is a completely disposable plastic urinal which folds flat and is therefore very easy to carry. It is useful for journeys and for those who suddenly get 'caught short' in public. The non-return valve and wire ties enable it to be carried after use until a suitable place is found for disposal. However, as it can only be used once (the non-return valve ensures that it must be cut to be emptied), it is too expensive for routine use, but good for special situations or locations.

The female swan-necked urinal (Figure 9.2(e)) is useful for men with a retracted penis who have difficulty in using a standard bottle. The whole penis and scrotum can usually fit inside the neck of the bottle, so that urine is caught at whatever angle it emerges.

Female hand-held urinals (Figure 9.3)

Women who cannot get to a lavatory or commode, or find sitting on one painful, have a variety of alternative urinals available. A standard hospital model bedpan can be used, although they tend to be rather large and cumbersome and are difficult to get onto without assistance. Many disabled people are too unstable to sit upright unaided on a bedpan, and these are very uncomfortable to use lying down. Smaller hand-held urinals tend to be easier to use independently, provided that the individual has reasonable manual dexterity.

Some women construct their own urinals from items such as household funnels, tubing and hot-water bottles. A narrow tall jug is useful if there is difficulty in abducting the thighs.

The pan-type female urinal (Figure 9.3(a), e.g. Suba Seal, Freeman) is a shallow plastic dish with a rounded lip for comfort and to prevent spillage. It is emptied via the rubber cap on the handle. It can be used in bed or on a chair. Women who cannot raise the buttocks to position it can often roll onto it sideways, as it is shallow. Someone who is bed-bound can empty it into a bucket by the bed and re-use it without assistance.

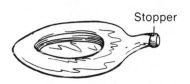

Stopper

Figure 9.3
Female hand-held urinals.

(a) Pan type urinal
(Suba Seal; Freeman)

The slipper bed-pan (Figure 9.3(b)) is similar in use to the Suba Seal, only larger.

The St Peter's Boat (Figure 9.3(c)) is a pear-shaped dish with a handle which can be used either on the edge of a bed or chair, with the knees apart, or standing up.

The Feminal (Figure 9.3(d), Franklin Medical) is designed to fit the female vulva closely and collect urine in a disposable plastic bag. Again, this may be used on the edge of a bed or chair, or when standing. Considerable dexterity is necessary to attach the plastic bag and to position the Feminal correctly for use. As it is small and light it is easy to carry on journeys. The plastic bag can be sealed with wire tags after use and put in a water-tight container until emptying is possible. The Feminal is not suitable for patients with very limited thigh abduction or impaired perineal sensation.

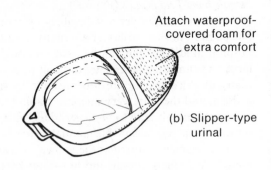

(b) Slipper-type urinal

(c) St Peters Boat

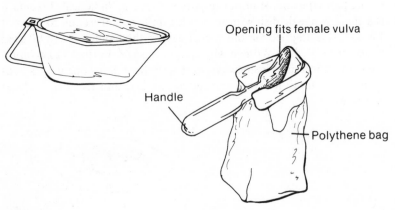

Figure 9.3
(continuation)

(d) Female urinal (Feminal; Franklin)

Women in wheelchairs may find hand-held urinals easier to use with a specially adapted cushion with a removable U-shaped cut-out in front which leaves a gap for the urinal (*Equipment for the Disabled*, 1984, p.47).

Neither men nor women will want to use a hand-held urinal in full public view. Sometimes a travel rug over the knees may be used to conceal what is happening. A hand-held urinal can enable the disabled person to undertake activities which would normally be impossible, such as visiting public places without lavatories for the disabled, or travelling by train. It is advisable to practise at home in private before trusting to their use in public.

CLOTHING

The disabled person can be aided in maintaining continence by the choice of suitable clothing.

Men with poor dexterity may find Velcro fly fastenings easier and quicker to undo than buttons or a zip. It is easier to use a bottle if the fly-opening is extended right down to the crotch seam (e.g. Edgware trousers, Figure 9.4(a)). Some men may find it easier to use loose-fitting boxer-style underpants rather than bikini briefs or Y-fronts.

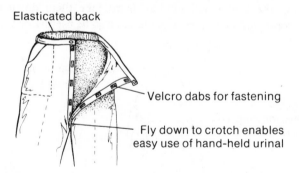

Elasticated back

Velcro dabs for fastening

Fly down to crotch enables easy use of hand-held urinal

Figure 9.4 *Adaptations to clothing.* (a) *Trousers with extended opening and Velcro fastening.*

Many women, especially older women, wear several layers of clothing (e.g. skirt, petticoat, corset, vest and pants). It can take considerable time and agility to get them out of the way, and accidental wetting or soiling is common. Tight skirts can be difficult to pull up in a hurry. People who have problems should be encouraged to wear loose clothing, and the fewer layers the better. Wrap-around skirts with a generous overlap are easy to pull onto the lap out of the way (Figure 9.4(b)).

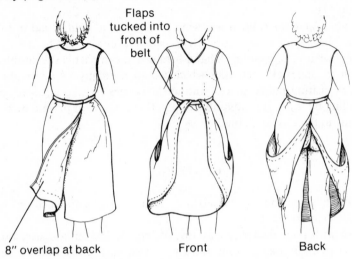

Figure 9.4 (b) *Wrap-around skirt.*

Women using hand-held urinals may find that split-crotch pants and tights, or loose French knickers, can be pulled out of the way when using the urinal without having to take them down (Figure 9.4(c)). Drop-front incontinence pants can also be useful (see Ch. 13).

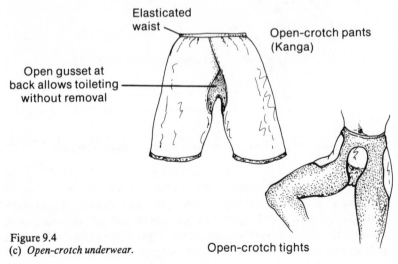

Figure 9.4
(c) *Open-crotch underwear.*

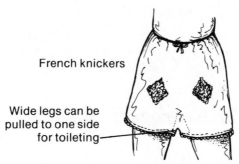

French knickers

Wide legs can be
pulled to one side
for toileting

Many physically disabled people can be helped to be continent either by adapting lavatories to their needs or by providing acceptable alternatives. Increased public awareness has led to the needs of the disabled being more often considered, but there is still a long way to go before facilities are universal. Detailed individual assessment will indicate the most suitable solution for each patient. In this assessment the nurse, occupational therapist and physiotherapist should ideally work together with the disabled person and his family to arrive at an answer.

In some areas an aids centre is run by the health authority or the social services department, or by a voluntary organisation. The disabled person, accompanied by a therapist, can receive expert assessment and help, and often try different aids before a decision is made to order an item.

REFERENCES AND FURTHER READING

Association of Continence Advisors, 1985. *Directory of Aids to Toileting*, London.

British Standards Institution, 1979. *Access for the Disabled to Buildings.* BS 5810:1979, BSI, London.

Disabled Living Foundation Information Service. Leaflet 7A (Personal Toilet); 7B (Personal Care), DLF, London.

Equipment for the Disabled, 1984. *The Management of Urinary and Faecal Incontinence and Stomata: A Guide for Health Professionals* (first edn.), Mary Marlborough Lodge, Nuffield Orthopaedic Centre, Oxford.

Goldsmith, S., 1976. *Designing for the Disabled* (3rd edn.), RIBA Publications, London.

Royal Association for Disability and Rehabilitation, 1984. *Access to Public Conveniences*, RADAR, London.

The following Patient Organisations provide information sheets for members (addresses in Appendix 2): Association for Spina Bifida and Hydrocephalus, Multiple Sclerosis Society, Sexual and Personal Relationships of the Disabled, Spinal Injuries Association.

Chapter 10

The Neurogenic Bladder

For many people with incontinence and other bladder problems the underlying cause is damage to the delicate neurological control mechanisms which regulate bladder function. As discussed in Chapter 2, continence is dependent on very long nerve pathways which are vulnerable to disease or trauma affecting the nervous system.

The problems of those with neurogenic bladder dysfunction are often exacerbated by the fact that bladder control is seldom the only impairment; many people will have varying degrees of physical and/or mental disability. When poor bladder function and disability co-exist, the problems involved in coping with micturition and incontinence are compounded. The specific problems associated with physical disabilities are dealt with in the previous chapter. The interaction of actual bladder problems and the physical ability to cope with them should be borne in mind throughout this chapter.

Damage to nerve pathways at any point between the cortical bladder centre and the bladder itself can impair continence. Dysfunction will depend upon the exact site and the extent of the lesion. Figure 10.1 illustrates the five possible sites of damage. It should be remembered that diffuse neurological disease such as multiple sclerosis, or multiple injuries, may cause any combination of these problems.

SITES OF NEUROLOGICAL DAMAGE

Cortical bladder centre

The higher cortical centres which control micturition may be involved in cerebrovascular accident, diffuse cortical failure and dementia, or multiple sclerosis, and may be damaged by a cerebral tumour or head injury. 'Normal' age-changes in the brain result in impairment of function in a high percentage of older people. Damage impairs the individual's ability to inhibit the sacral reflex arc efficiently (see Figure 2.2). In many cases bladder sensation is retained so that urgency is felt,

174

The Neurogenic Bladder

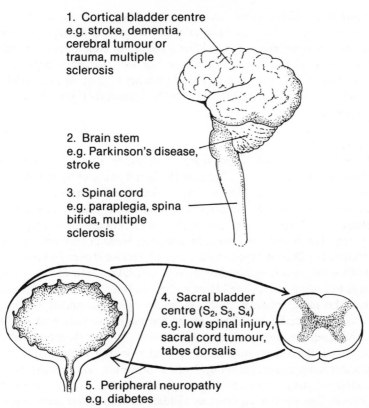

1. Cortical bladder centre
e.g. stroke, dementia,
cerebral tumour or
trauma, multiple
sclerosis

2. Brain stem
e.g. Parkinson's disease,
stroke

3. Spinal cord
e.g. paraplegia, spina
bifida, multiple
sclerosis

4. Sacral bladder
centre (S_2, S_3, S_4)
e.g. low spinal injury,
sacral cord tumour,
tabes dorsalis

5. Peripheral neuropathy
e.g. diabetes

Figure 10.1 *Sites of neurological damage leading to neurogenic bladder problems.*

but the all-important inhibiting signal is weak or absent, and urgency and urge incontinence may result. This condition is identical to detrusor instability (see Chapter 2), and the term 'unstable bladder' can be used to describe an uninhibited bladder whether of neurogenic or idiopathic origin.

Brain stem
Centres in the brain stem are vital in co-ordinating the complex series of reflexes and feedback loops involved in the act of complete voluntary micturition. Damage (e.g. in Parkinson's disease, multiple sclerosis, some dementias) will result in a poorly co-ordinated and often incomplete voiding sequence. Normally, during micturition the detrusor should contract and the urethra relax synergically, functioning

175

together to effect rapid and complete bladder emptying without interruption, straining or residual urine. Brain stem damage can result in detrusor-sphincter dyssynergia – the sphincter does not relax adequately as the detrusor contracts, or the bladder contraction is unsustained. This may result in total inability to void, or in all voiding being by abdominal effort only, or in interrupted and incomplete emptying.

Spinal cord

Complete transection of the spinal cord above the level of the sacral bladder centre usually results, after the initial phase of 'spinal shock' is over, in an 'automatic' bladder that is decentralised from all cerebral control. Immediately after spinal injury most people experience a phase of 'silence' during which all spinal reflexes are disrupted or absent. The bladder is completely atonic, without any activity, and retention of urine is experienced. Once this phase is over and the spinal reflexes become re-established (which can take anything from a few days to several years), the bladder starts to 'wake up' again. Provided that the sacral bladder centre is undamaged, the spinal reflex arc becomes re-established. The patient has neither sensation of bladder activity nor any control over reflex contractions. As the bladder is cut off from the reflex co-ordinating centre in the brain stem, these bladder contractions, although often powerful, are frequently not sustained, and incomplete emptying with residual urine is often also present. The patient experiences sudden uncontrollable incontinence, but this does not always leave an empty bladder.

If transection is incomplete, some conscious sensation and some voluntary control may be retained.

Sacral bladder centre

If spinal-cord damage involves sacral segments S_2–S_4, the spinal reflex arc will be disrupted. There will be neither conscious sensation nor voluntary control of the bladder, and the detrusor contraction reflex will be absent. The bladder is atonic in response to filling, although it is possible that local synapses in the bladder wall may cause minor ineffectual contractions. This atonic bladder will become increasingly distended and overflow incontinence usually develops. Any bladder emptying will be by abdominal effort alone.

This type of bladder was once commonly seen in tabes dorsalis of tertiary syphilis. Those with low spinal injury or tumour and spina bifida are the most common sufferers today.

Peripheral neuropathy
Disease of the peripheral nervous system can attack the local nerve supply to the bladder. This is especially common in diabetic peripheral neuropathy, which can affect both sensory and motor pathways. Because sensation is deficient the bladder may be allowed to become overdistended. Motor damage leads to inefficient bladder emptying, and overflow incontinence may develop. Extensive pelvic surgery may likewise disrupt peripheral nerves.

As will be seen from the above, neurogenic bladder problems fall into two broad categories of dysfunction: those resulting in an unstable or uninhibited bladder (e.g. cortical or spinal damage), and those causing voiding problems (brain stem, spinal, sacral, or peripheral damage). Even where these two co-exist they should usually be managed as two distinct entities and treated separately.

INVESTIGATIONS

Neurogenic bladder problems should always be fully investigated prior to treatment. Urodynamic investigations are essential to accurate pinpointing of the problem. A cystometrogram (Chapter 3) should be done with a much slower fill-rate than normal (e.g. 10ml per minute instead of 60–100ml), as too fast a fill may provoke the bladder into bizarre activity. Where voiding difficulties are suspected, X-ray facilities are helpful as the bladder neck and urethra can be visualised during attempted voiding (videocystourethrography). Electro-myelogram (EMG) recordings may help diagnosis of dyssynergic sphincter activity.

If the patient is disabled, a careful assessment of mobility, dexterity, and life-style will also be vital in planning a realistic goal for each individual (see Chapters 3 and 9).

MANAGEMENT

MANAGEMENT OF THE UNSTABLE NEUROGENIC BLADDER

This is very similar to management of detrusor instability of non-neurogenic origin (see Chapter 4). The uninhibited contractions can often be damped down, even eliminated, by drug therapy. Care must be taken with patients with neuropathy, as a few are hypersensitive to medication and may be tipped into retention or experience exaggerated side-effects, especially from anticholinergic therapy. For this reason new treatments should be introduced gradually and monitored closely.

Accurate charting will reveal whether there is a pattern to the instability and incontinence. If the volume of bladder filling at which contractions occur is relatively constant, it is often possible to plan a toileting programme designed to anticipate incontinence. This will obviously vary with fluid intake and may need to take activities into account, as movement may provoke bladder contractions. The role of bladder training has not been well evaluated in this group but it is likely to be effective in some cases (see Chapter 4 for method).

Many people with an unstable neurogenic bladder have considerably restricted mobility (for instance, after a stroke or spinal injury). This greatly adds to the problem of managing a bladder which is unpredictable and gives minimal, if any, warning of impending incontinence.

MANAGEMENT OF NEUROGENIC VOIDING DIFFICULTIES

Incomplete bladder-emptying can lead to a number of problems. Urinary tract infection is common if residual urine is present and, because the bladder is never completely emptied, is extremely difficult to eradicate, even with antibiotics. Re-infection and a shifting spectrum of invading organisms are common. If the residual volume is large, in particular over 400ml, there is some risk of renal damage from back-pressure via the ureters. If hydronephrosis is present, with or without ureteric reflux, renal infection usually follows bladder infection. This carries a high risk of morbidity and possible mortality.

Residual urine also often leads to overflow incontinence. It also reduces functional bladder capacity. (If the bladder capacity is 500ml, with a residual urine volume of 400ml, the functional capacity – that capacity which can be used – is only 100ml.) This will obviously increase voiding frequency considerably. Those who have the double problem of a residual volume and instability (e.g. some people with multiple sclerosis or spinal injury) often only have a very small margin between their residual volume, which is always in the bladder, and the volume at which uninhibited contractions develop. This can result in incontinence occurring very soon after voiding. Indeed, some will suffer almost continuous episodes of incontinence, since as soon as the volume in the bladder exceeds the residual volume the bladder contracts and expels the excess.

Voiding techniques
Some people with a voiding difficulty manage to find a technique that will stimulate complete voiding.

If the elements of the sacral reflex are intact but merely unco-ordinated (e.g. cut off from the brain stem) it is often possible voluntarily to initiate a detrusor contraction by stimulation of trigger areas. Alternatively, direct rises in abdominal pressure, especially in women, can raise intravesical pressure to the point where urethral resistance is overcome and voluntary voiding occurs (Valsalva or Crede manoeuvres). If either of these can be done before overflow incontinence occurs, with the individual appropriately placed over a receptacle, continence can be achieved.

Trigger areas. Patients without sacral damage may find a 'trigger' that will initiate a bladder contraction. Tapping the abdominal wall suprapubically is a common method. The abdomen is firmly and repeatedly tapped, usually by the tips of extended fingers of one hand, until voiding starts. Often the contraction generated is unsustained, so the tapping and voiding has to be repeated several times until the bladder is empty. Abdominal tenderness or weak fingers may be a problem. If the reflex is weak, a long period of tapping may be required before micturition starts, and it may have to be frequently repeated before the bladder is completely empty. It can therefore become very time-consuming and demoralising. However, because bladder contraction usually initiates some urethral opening, the potential for damage is low, and this method is preferable to straining, or pushing, for those who can achieve it.

Other trigger areas that work for some people are pulling pubic hairs, stroking the abdomen or interior aspect of the thighs, or digital anal stimulation and dilation (Johnson, 1980). Patients managing their voiding difficulties in this way should experiment to discover which area works best and most easily for them.

Valsalva and Crede. Both of these techniques are only suitable for those whose sphincter mechanism is not in complete spasm: usually patients with damage at the sacral bladder centre level, when sphincteric resistance is often low and easily overcome.

The Valsalva manoeuvre (inhaling deeply and then exhaling force-fully against a closed glottis) greatly increases intra-abdominal pressure and may enable bladder emptying by straining. Alternatively, in some people this pressure rise may trigger a bladder contraction. However, this type of straining is inadvisable, certainly on a long-term regular basis. It raises intra-cranial pressure and impedes cardiac return, and should definitely be avoided by anyone with cardiovascular or cerebrovascular disease. Straining may eventually weaken and damage pelvic floor musculature and the bladder neck, leading to sphincter incompetence (stress incontinence).

The Crede manoeuvre, or manual bladder expression, involves applying considerable pressure, usually with the ball of the hand or a fist, suprapubically directly over the bladder. Like Valsalva, this may work to empty the bladder either by directly raising bladder pressure or by triggering a contraction. Unfortunately, if no contraction occurs the bladder neck will remain closed, and a very high pressure is needed to overcome this; eventual sphincter damage is a risk. Some people find expression uncomfortable. If sensation is deficient, great care should be taken to avoid bruising. Obese people and those with weak hands or arms also have difficulty. Sometimes someone else can be taught to apply the pressure. If reflux is suspected from the bladder to the ureters the Crede manoeuvre should be avoided. Whether its repeated use can create reflux is unproven.

Intermittent catheterisation

There can be little doubt that the biggest single advance that has been made in the management of neurogenic voiding difficulties has been the introduction of intermittent catheterisation. This involves the episodic introduction of a catheter into the bladder to remove any residual urine, and then removal of the catheter, leaving the patient catheter-free between catheterisations.

Sterile intermittent catheterisation was originally introduced for the immediate post-injury management of patients with a spinal injury. A strictly aseptic technique is used and the procedure is performed by a doctor or nurse at intervals sufficiently frequent to keep the residual volume below 400ml. This procedure was introduced as an alternative to using an indwelling catheter in the phase of spinal shock, when the bladder is areflexic. There is considerably less risk of infection and complications than with a permanent indwelling catheter, and a better long-term prognosis in terms of catheter-free continence.

In hospital, or anywhere where a catheterisation is being done by a doctor or nurse, risks of cross-infection are high and it is always best to maintain a strict aseptic policy. For single use a Jacques or Nelaton plastic catheter, size 10 or 12 f.g., is the best and cheapest (Fig. 10.2).

In the past decade, the technique of intermittent non-sterile ('clean') self-catheterisation has become widely adopted for the long-term

The Neurogenic Bladder

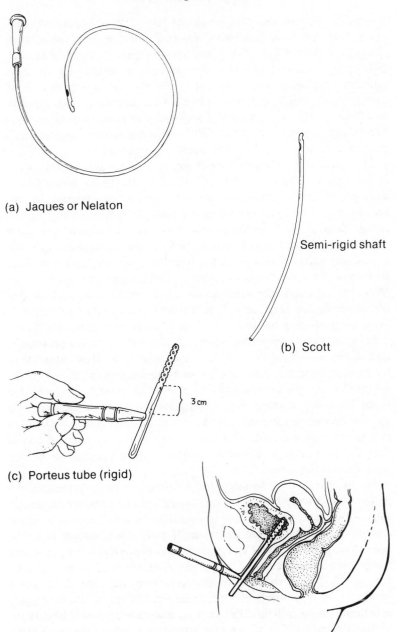

Figure 10.2 *Catheters suitable for intermittent catheterisation.*

181

management of people with persistent large residual urine volumes. Most work has been done with children suffering from spina bifida (Kaye and Van Blerk, 1981) and spinal-injury patients (Pearman, 1976), whose spinal shock does not resolve sufficiently to leave efficient voiding reflexes. More recently its use has spread to all categories of people with incomplete bladder emptying. Many people of all ages, both sexes, and with a wide range of physical abilities, have been taught to self-catheterise. Where this has proved impossible, a relative or regular carer has often been taught instead.

The clean technique was introduced by Lapides and his colleagues in the USA in the early 1970s (Lapides et al., 1972). Much to the surprise of many professionals brought up on theories of the importance of strict asepsis in catheterisation, patients using a clean rather than a sterile technique do not tend to encounter frequent problematic urinary tract infection. In fact, many who previously had chronically infected residual urine find that infection decreases from its former incidence when intermittent catheterisation is used, as the focus for infection (the residual urine) is removed. It is likely that complete regular emptying of the bladder is an important factor in preventing infection becoming established in the urinary tract.

Many nurses are perturbed when they first encounter this procedure, and worry about infection risks (especially with clean rather than sterile intermittent catheterisation) and the dangers of trauma to the urethra from repeated catheter insertions. In practice the risks are slight (certainly nothing approaching the problems associated with indwelling catheterisation), and very few patients have to abandon intermittent catheterisation because of problems, provided of course that the procedure is correctly taught and the programme closely supervised in the initial stages.

To be selected as suitable for intermittent catheterisation, the patient will usually have a residual urine volume persistently greater than 100ml, and be experiencing problems of overflow incontinence and/or recurrent bladder infection. If self-catheterisation is to be successful, a reasonable degree of manual dexterity, intelligence and motivation are necessary. The parents or teachers of young children are usually taught to perform the technique until the child is old enough to be responsible himself, usually at the age of seven or eight, depending on the individual's character and developmental level (Fay, 1978). A close relative or constant attendant may be able and willing to learn to help the disabled adult who cannot manage self-catheterisation. Before this option is considered, it must be ensured that it would be acceptable to both patient and relative, and that the relationship between them would not be unduly stressed by this additional dependence.

The technique of intermittent catheterisation should be fully discussed with the patient as a preliminary to teaching the method. Many patients are worried at the idea of using a catheter initially, and will wish to discuss the possibilities of causing damage to themselves and what the long-term effects will be. A few, especially women, are embarrassed at the idea of touching the genitals and (rarely) some people reject the technique completely for this reason. It is important that whoever is teaching the patient, whether nurse or doctor, approaches the subject in a very down-to-earth fashion, imparting optimism that the patient will both be able to do it and will benefit. The alternatives, including voiding techniques, indwelling catheter, surgery or drugs, and continuing with the voiding difficulty and overflow incontinence, should be outlined, with the advantages and disadvantages of each. For many patients, intermittent self-catheterisation is the treatment of choice and should be strongly recommended by professionals. However, this will not be successful without the patient's full and intelligent co-operation and cannot be started unless the patient is willing.

People vary greatly in their aptitude for self-catheterisation. Teaching should always take place in a relaxed, private and unhurried environment. If several different members of staff are involved with the patient it is a good idea to have a written, consistent policy, so that he is told the same thing by everyone. Firstly a full and detailed explanation of the local anatomy is given, usually with the aid of diagrams (Figure 10.3, overleaf). Few people have an accurate idea of important facts such as the length of the urethra, or the relationship of the various genital organs. Many have fears: for example, that the catheter might get lost inside or that they could puncture the bladder if the catheter goes in too far. The patient is then catheterised in the semi-recumbent position and a detailed commentary given. Usually the teacher (doctor or nurse) should be using asepsis (because of the risk of cross-infection), and it must be explained to the patient why a clean technique is adequate for the patient's use outside hospital. Most people will understand an explanation that everyone has a certain resistance to his own bacteria, and as the bladder will be completely and regularly emptied, any bacteria which are introduced will be drained out again and so cannot take hold. The nurse (or doctor) must wear gloves and take extra precautions to protect the patient from the bacteria of other patients and of the nurse herself.

Once the catheter is in position, women should be shown the position of the urethral meatus in a mirror, and locate by hand how far it is from an easily identifiable landmark (e.g. the clitoris or labia). The woman should then withdraw the catheter herself, and re-introduce it by parting the labia with the non-dominant hand and locating the meatus in a mirror. With a little practice most women can learn to self-catheterise by touch (indeed, some never manage to get a reasonable view in the mirror), which is an advantage as the mirror can then be dispensed with. Having successfully introduced the catheter two or

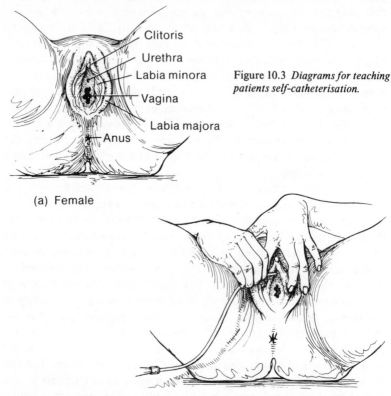

Clitoris

Urethra

Labia minora

Vagina

Labia majora

Anus

Figure 10.3 *Diagrams for teaching patients self-catheterisation.*

(a) Female

three times lying down with the legs abducted, the patient is then asked to catheterise sitting on a lavatory, by touch if possible. If a mirror is needed, a shaving mirror may be adapted to hook over the front of the lavatory seat, or a suction pad attached to the seat or front of the bowl. Some women cannot manage this, and indeed there are a variety of positions which may suit individual preferences or disabilities.

Squatting, standing with one foot on a stool or lavatory pan, sitting on the edge of a chair or wheelchair (with a U cut-out cushion if necessary, see page 171), or using a posterior approach if the legs cannot be abducted, may all be found suitable, depending upon the patient's physical abilities and agility.

Male patients naturally have far less difficulty than females in locating the urethral meatus, and may self-catheterise lying, sitting, or standing, as convenient. Most men use lignocaine gel inserted into the urethra prior to inserting the catheter. Some women also prefer to use a little gel either into the urethra or on the catheter.

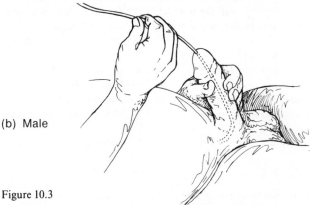

(b) Male

Figure 10.3

Many people learn to self-catheterise competently in a single out-patient session. Others will be in hospital anyway, and some outpatients may benefit from a few days in hospital to perfect the technique under supervision. Very handicapped people may take considerably longer to find a position and method that is reliable. Some women with limited movement in the hand and wrist may find a Porteus tube easier than a soft plastic catheter, or a shorter, more rigid Scott catheter (see Figure 10.2).

Frequency of catheterisation will vary with individual needs. Some people almost empty the bladder at micturition, and have a residual urine which slowly accumulates over a few days. Others are in complete retention and will need to catheterise five to six times a day. It should be done often enough to avoid incontinence wherever possible, as well as to ensure that the volume of residual urine obtained is always below 400ml. Once the technique is mastered the patient may be sent away with an adequate supply of catheters and a simple instruction sheet and diagram (Tables 10.1 & 10.2, overleaf, and Figure 10.3).

Table 10.1: Self-Catheterisation for Women

1) Perform the catheterisation as often as your doctor or nurse has suggested. To start with, this should be every . . . hours.
2) Get your catheter, a mirror, and lubricant gel if you need it.
3) Wash your hands – thoroughly – and rinse the catheter under the tap.
4) Position yourself in the most comfortable and convenient position. If you do not sit on the lavatory, you will need a jug or receiver for the urine.
5) Part the labia with one hand and, holding the catheter 2–3 inches from the tip, gently insert it into the urethra until urine flows (see diagram).
6) When urine stops flowing, slowly withdraw the catheter. If the flow re-starts, stop withdrawing until the bladder is empty. It is most important that the bladder is completely emptied at each catheterisation.
7) When the catheter is out, wash it with a mild solution of washing-up liquid, rinse it thoroughly, and shake it dry. Dry the outside with a clean paper towel or tissue and store it in a clean dry place ready for the next use. If you are keeping a chart, record the urine volume obtained.
8) Use each catheter for one week and then throw it away and use a new one. A supply of catheters is available from the hospital or from your own doctor on prescription.
9) You should drink 3–4 pints of liquid (any type) every twenty-four hours.

What should I do if . . .?

. . . I see blood in the urine or on the catheter?
If this is a few specks, don't worry. If the bleeding persists or becomes heavy, contact the clinic.

. . . the urine becomes smelly, cloudy, or if burning or a fever develop?
Bring a urine specimen up to the clinic. You probably have a mild infection.

. . . I cannot get the catheter in?
Don't keep trying, you will get sore. Abandon the attempt and try again later. If the difficulty persists and you are unable to pass urine yourself, seek help within twelve hours.

. . . I miss and put the catheter in the vagina?
You will know because it will feel different and no urine will come out. Take the catheter out, wash it and start again.

Clinic telephone no: .... (Hours ....)
In an emergency contact your own general practitioner.

Table 10.2: Self-Catheterisation for Men

1) Perform the catheterisation as often as your doctor or nurse has suggested. To start with this should be every . . . hours.
2) Get your catheter and lubricant gel.
3) Wash your hands – thoroughly – and rinse the catheter under the tap.
4) Position yourself in the most comfortable and convenient position. If you do not sit on the lavatory, you will need a jug or receiver for the urine.
5) If you need to use anaesthetic gel, insert this into the tip of the penis, holding the penis slightly erect, then pinch gently to retain the gel. Wait four minutes for anaesthetic to take effect.
6) If you do not need anaesthetic gel, squeeze a small amount of lubricant gel along the catheter.
7) Holding the penis in a vertical position, gently insert the catheter until urine flows (see diagram). You may find that pretending to pass urine or coughing helps overcome any resistance at the sphincter.
8) When urine stops flowing, slowly withdraw the catheter. If the flow re-starts, stop withdrawing until the bladder is empty. It is most important that the bladder is completely emptied at each catheterisation.
9) When the catheter is out, wash it with a mild solution of washing-up liquid, rinse it thoroughly, and shake it dry. Dry the outside with a clean paper towel or tissue and store it in a clean dry place ready for the next use. If you are keeping a chart, record the urine volume obtained.
10) Use each catheter for one week and then throw it away and use a new one. A supply of catheters is available from the hospital or from your own doctor on prescription.
11) You should drink 3–4 pints of liquid (any type) every twenty-four hours.

What should I do if . . .?

. . . I see blood in the urine or on the catheter?
If this is a few specks don't worry. If the bleeding persists or becomes heavy, contact the clinic.

. . . the urine becomes smelly, cloudy, or if burning or a fever develop?
Bring a urine specimen up to the clinic. You probably have a mild infection.

. . . I cannot get the catheter in?
Don't keep trying, you will get sore. Abandon the attempt and try again later. If the difficulty persists and you are unable to pass urine yourself, seek help within twelve hours.

Clinic telephone no: .... (Hours ....)
In an emergency contact your own general practitioner.

At home, each catheter is washed out after use (e.g. with a mild solution of washing-up liquid), rinsed in running water and dried (shaken and the outside wiped with a paper towel). It is then stored in a clean dry place until next use, when it should again be held under a running tap prior to insertion. Many people use snap-sealing plastic bags to keep the catheter in a handbag or pocket between uses. Soaking the catheter in strong antiseptic solutions is usually discouraged as unnecessary. It may also possibly be irritant to the sensitive urethral mucosa and also have the potential to kill off normal flora, leaving the patient vulnerable to more harmful micro-organisms. Likewise, swabbing of the urethral meatus is not encouraged unless a discharge or vaginal infection is present. Each catheter is used for approximately one week and then thrown away (except in hospital, where a new catheter must be used each time to avoid cross-infection risks).

The importance of hand-washing is stressed to the patient. Women are instructed simply to wash their hands, part the labia, and insert the catheter until urine flows. Once the flow ceases the catheter is withdrawn slowly, halting if the flow starts again. Men do exactly the same, using lignocaine gel in addition when inserting the catheter, as already mentioned.

Significant infection, when the patient is unwell, feverish and has pain, offensive urine or haematuria, is relatively uncommon. It will occur in one-quarter to one-third of patients at some time. It will usually respond to single-dose trimethoprim (400mg nocte), since most infections are *E.coli* from gut contamination. If there are recurrent episodes it may be advisable to give the patient a small supply of trimethoprim to take when needed. A urine specimen should be cultured if symptoms fail to respond. Recurrent infection becomes a problem with a small minority of patients, and in this case the patient should be observed for any fault in technique. The volumes obtained should be measured to ensure that they are consistently below 400ml (infection results more often from catheterising too infrequently than from too frequently: Champion, 1976). Occasionally it is necessary to advise sterilising the catheters or changing them more frequently. Only in rare cases does self-catheterisation have to be abandoned.

Asymptomatic bacteriuria is probably quite common in people self-catheterising (*Lancet*, 1979). Generally, unless the patient has vesico-ureteric reflux or is very young (under five years old) this does not matter and should be left untreated. Indeed, there is little point in obtaining routine urine samples. A sample is only indicated in the presence of symptoms. Treating asymptomatic infection predisposes to the development of more serious or resistant infection, and there is no benefit from eradicating a symptomless bacteriuria.

Where a patient has the dual problems of residual urine and unstable contractions, the aim of therapy should be to paralyse the bladder pharmacologically to abolish the contractions, and then to drain the bladder by intermittent catheterisation. This works well for many people with spina bifida, multiple sclerosis, or paraplegia.

The results from intermittent catheterisation are excellent. Up to 80% of patients with large-volume residual urine of neurogenic origin can regain continence. Many have thereby avoided a permanent indwelling catheter, with all its attendant problems (see Chapter 15), or a urinary diversion by ileal conduit. Some people can gradually phase out catheterisation as normal voiding is re-established. Others must continue to catheterise indefinitely. The procedure is too new to be able to say with confidence what the long-term prospects are, but certainly at present they look very hopeful. Indeed, some people with ileal conduits are now being 'undiverted' back to using their own bladder with intermittent catheterisation. The technique is also being increasingly used with elderly patients with a voiding difficulty (see Chapter 8).

Drug therapy
Various drug regimes may be used to assist voiding. Some drugs act by increasing the contractile power of an atonic bladder (e.g. bethanechol or carbachol). Others reduce outflow resistance (e.g. phenoxybenzamine or diazepam). All of them have significant side-effects and should be used with great care.

Surgery
In the past many males with neurogenic voiding difficulties had their urinary sphincters transected, thereby creating total incontinence, in order to preserve renal function. Today surgical techniques are more selective. A careful bladder-neck incision or resection or a urethrotomy may decrease outflow resistance to the point where a voiding technique can be effective, without necessarily creating incontinence. As men are not dependent on the internal sphincter for continence this can safely be resected and continence retained in some cases. However, many quadriplegic and some paraplegic men do become incontinent because of surgery to preserve renal function, and use penile sheath drainage on a long-term basis.

A urinary diversion by ileal conduit into a stoma should be a last resort in the management of neurogenic incontinence. It involves major surgery and the long-term prognosis for renal function is uncertain. However, if all else fails to restore continence, especially if renal function is threatened by recurrent infection, it should be seriously considered as an alternative to using an indwelling catheter (see Chapter 15), especially for women, for whom there is no satisfactory external collection device. Adjustment to surgery can be excellent with careful pre-operative counselling, and certainly an incontinent stoma is much easier to manage effectively than a totally incontinent female urethra. Where there seems little prospect of continence, a stoma may be offered to the patient relatively early, rather than waiting until she has endured years of misery and incontinence. Counselling from a stoma care nurse, where available, can help the patient and family to reach an informed decision.

MANAGEMENT OF THE BLADDER AFTER SPINAL INJURY

It is crucial for the eventual rehabilitation of the paraplegic patient and his bladder that good bladder management is started immediately after injury. Initially the patient will be in spinal shock with complete retention. If the bladder is allowed to become over-distended at this time, permanent progressive damage can be caused to the local nerve supply. Intermittent sterile catheterisation should be started immediately upon admission and a very careful record kept to ensure that the bladder is never allowed to hold more than 400ml of urine.

Very soon after injury, often within a few days (depending obviously upon his general health), the patient is encouraged to participate in his own bladder management. As soon as he is able to do so he is taught to self-catheterise and keep his own charts.

After a variable length of time the bladder starts to 'wake up' and reflex contractions start to occur. These will be inefficient at first and a decision must be made on individual criteria whether to augment these contractions by drugs or by tapping to achieve voiding, or else to suppress them pharmacologically and continue intermittent catheterisation.

The paraplegic, having either deficient or completely absent direct bladder sensation, can often learn to be very sensitive to other stimuli which help to monitor bladder fullness and activity. Some have autonomic cues when the bladder is full (commonly tachycardia but often other quite individual signs). Others can feel by the abdominal distension or by effects on the gut. It is most important that the patient learns to interpret these internal signals correctly as they greatly help in achieving continence. Nursing spinal injury patients should involve prolonged teaching sessions from an early stage.

In men, an unstable bladder with dyssynergic voiding is often the eventual outcome. This sphincter resistance is useful in maintaining continence but may need to be modified by drugs or surgery if voiding difficulty is significant. Alternatively, intermittent catheterisation may be continued.

Women often fare less well than men. Serious incontinence often results because the sphincter is so much less efficient once the reflexes are re-established. Drug therapy will sometimes dampen these contractions, but for some women incontinence may be so severe that urinary diversion is considered.

REFERENCES AND FURTHER READING

Barry, K., 1981. 'Neurogenic bladder incontinence: the consequences of mismanagement'. *Rehabilitation Nursing*, 10, 12–13.

Champion, V. L., 1976. 'Clean technique for intermittent self-catheterisation'. *Nursing Research*, 25, 1, 13–18.

Fay, J., 1978. 'Intermittent non-sterile catheterisation of children'. *Nursing Mirror*, 146, 14, xiii–xv.

Hartman, M., 1978. 'Intermittent self-catheterisation'. *Nursing 78*, 11, 72–75.

Holland, N. J., Wiesel-Levison, P., Schwedelson, E. S., 1981. 'Survey of neurogenic bladder in multiple sclerosis'. *Journal of Neurosurgical Nursing*, 13, 6, 337–343.

Johnson, J. H., 1980. 'Rehabilitative aspects of neurologic bladder dysfunction'. *Nursing Clinics of North America*, 15, 2, 293–307.

Kaye, K., Van Blerk, P. J. P., 1981. 'Urinary continence in children with neurogenic bladders'. *British Journal of Urology*, 53, 241–245.

Lancet, 1979. 'Clean intermittent catheterisation'., Vol. 2, 448–449.

Lapides, J., Diokno, A. C., Silber, S. J., Lowe, B. S., 1972. 'Clean intermittent self-catheterisation in the treatment of urinary tract disease'. *Journal of Urology*, 107, 458–461.

Pearman, J. W., 1976. 'Urological follow-up of 99 spinal-cord injured patients initially managed by intermittent catheterisation'. *British Journal of Urology*, 48, 297–310.

Spiro, L. R., 1978. 'Bladder training for the incontinent patient'. *Journal of Gerontological Nursing*, 4, 3, 28–35.

Chapter 11

Factors Related to Location

Wherever the incontinent person is, problems may be inherent in that location. This is true in an acute or long-stay hospital, residential or sheltered accommodation, or in his own or a relative's home. At times these location-related factors may cause or exacerbate incontinence, or at least work against successful cure or management.

HOME CARE

Few nurses who have worked exclusively in hospital realise just how different problems can be when experienced by the individual in his own home. The vast majority of incontinent people live at home. Most cope with their incontinence, often remarkably well, and manage to control the problem so that it creates only minimal disruption to their lives. At best, there may be just a little extra laundry or more items for disposal. But where incontinence is very heavy and poorly managed, it can become such a burden that it dominates home life, eventually leading to a breakdown of the ability to live independently or to be maintained at home by carers. Success in managing heavy incontinence at home will depend on who is available and their willingness to help, what washing and disposal facilities there are and which services can be mobilised to assist.

Assessment at home

Assessment of the incontinent person in his own environment is certainly desirable, and a home assessment will give the nurse a much clearer picture of the problem than could be obtained in a hospital clinic. However, assessment at home may also involve problems. The nurse, as a guest in the home, is often less in control of the situation than she is in hospital, and some people, the lonely elderly especially, may be very difficult to keep to the point of the discussion. The interview invariably takes longer, and it is important to allow plenty of time when planning an assessment visit. Some people deny their incontinence when visited at home. If the patient does not live alone it may be difficult to ensure privacy, and he may be unwilling to talk frankly in front of others, whether children, parents, or spouse.

Physical examination is more difficult in many homes. The bedroom may be cold and poorly lit, and a vulval inspection may be almost impossible on a sagging mattress in a dim light. Some people object to being examined at all. Any specimens obtained, such as a MSSU, will be less fresh by the time they get to the laboratory than a clinic specimen would be.

Unlike the assessment of patients in hospital, the home assessment is based on a short period of observation only. If the patient was expecting the visit, a special effort may have been made to tidy up, to hide the real effect that incontinence is having upon the home. Sometimes several visits are necessary both to gain the patient's full confidence and to build up a true picture of the problem.

Many people being visited by a community nurse or health visitor are suffering incontinence without the nurse realising it. The alert nurse, whether visiting to dress a leg ulcer or to do a development check on a child, will use her relationship with the patient to discover any other health-care problems, including incontinence, and to take appropriate action if necessary. A mutual pretence that incontinence is not occurring – denial by the patient or failure to enquire by the nurse – will reinforce the myth that incontinence is inevitable and untreatable, thereby missing the opportunity of remedy before the condition progresses. It is the nurse's responsibility to use every chance to promote optimum health for all her clients or patients.

Discharge from hospital
When an incontinent person is to be discharged from hospital, successful transition to coping at home will often depend on careful planning and liaison between hospital and community services. Rehabilitation in hospital must be geared to the realities of the home circumstances. Because someone can cope with incontinence in hospital, in a purpose-built environment with ample availability of aids and help, this does not necessarily mean he can cope as well at home.

Unfortunately, communications are often deficient. All too often people are sent home with inadequate preparation and without the new carers being informed of the full picture. Plenty of notice will be required, particularly if home modifications are needed, but also to arrange services such as home help, laundry, or bath nurse. The patient should have been taught in hospital how to use the aids which will be available in the home, and continuity of supplies is essential. People are often sent home with only a few days' supply of pads or appliances and with no guidance on where to get more. The nurse should have taught the patient, or his relatives, how to cope with problems like skin care, and advised on practical management at home, prior to discharge. To do this, the hospital nurse needs to be fully aware of the difficulties that are likely to be encountered in the home.

Self-care

Those with a limited capacity for self-care are often vulnerable at home. Many bowel problems are caused by constipation arising from a poor diet. This may be because of the high cost of fresh food, or the inability to shop or to cook, or the lack of motivation to prepare meals, especially for one person on his or her own. Those who receive meals-on-wheels may find them unpalatable, or cold. Some meals are delivered too early, when the recipient does not feel like eating. Some people are unable even to make themselves a drink, and become very dehydrated at home. This will aggravate any bowel or bladder problems and may, in extreme cases, lead to a confusional state.

Personal hygiene may be a problem for some people at home. The incontinent need to be especially scrupulous to avoid skin problems and odour, and where the individual cannot manage effectively, he is dependent on the home nursing service to perform these tasks for him.

Carers at home

In a hospital, however short of staff, there is always someone around for twenty-four hours in the day. This means that it should, in theory, be possible to gear toileting times to the individual's requirements. This is crucial if help is needed in getting to or onto the lavatory or in using a urinal. Someone who is not completely self-sufficient in toileting is dependent on others, and the availability of help at the required time will often determine whether or not incontinence occurs. Once wet, those with impaired physical or mental function may be unable to deal with the consequences independently and may be obliged to stay wet until help arrives. Dependence on others ranges from needing a verbal prompt to remind the forgetful that it is time to visit the lavatory, to needing help to rise from a chair, to requiring bodily transportation and lifting onto the lavatory.

However, the heavily incontinent person may live alone. Others may live with someone who is just as (or even more) forgetful or frail. Many more are alone for at least part of the day. If dependence is total and the bladder unpredictable (as may be the case with urge incontinence), continence is unlikely without constant attendance. If incontinence does occur, the longer the time lapse between wetting and changing, the greater the likelihood of discomfort, skin problems and odour. Some disabled people are incontinent, even if their bladder function is normal, simply because no one is available to help when needed. Many district nurses will have come across people living alone who are virtually helpless between the visits of the morning and evening nurse. Very few bladders are capable of reliably holding urine for twelve hours or more, and sooner or later voluntary wetting is inevitable. In some such cases it is possible with forethought and planning to organise a system to enable toilet visits at intervals throughout the day (e.g. spacing out the visits of the district nurse, home help, good neighbour, etc.), but this is unrealistic for many people. Others may manage with a hand-held urinal (see Chapter 9), but many women cannot manage this alone. Every effort should be made to avoid the degrading situation where an individual is obliged to pass urine onto the bed or chair because there is no help to hand. Some disabled incontinent people may qualify for Attendance Allowance if in need of 'frequent attention in connection with bodily functions'. This is a non-means-tested benefit, paid at a lower rate for day or night attendance, or at a higher rate if constant attendance is needed. The money may be used to help with the cost of a live-in or non-resident carer, and should be claimed via the local social security office. If a carer of working age is unable to work because he is looking after a disabled relative or friend who is receiving Attendance Allowance, he may be entitled to Invalid Care Allowance, provided that care is given for at least thirty-five hours per week. Married women do not qualify for this benefit.

Even when someone is available it is not always easy to transfer a disabled person onto the lavatory. In hospital two nurses may manage easily, but a frail spouse may be unable to cope. Good instructions may help a carer to learn lifting techniques, and the nurse must take care that faulty methods do not put the carer himself at risk of injury or disability. Often a well co-ordinated set of aids will facilitate transfer – for example, a bed, commode and wheelchair all at the same height and with detachable arms for sideways transfer, or an electric hoist, if appropriate.

The help that is available may be unacceptable, either to the patient or to the carer. Many elderly people are embarrassed for their spouse to aid with toileting, especially to assist in the more intimate tasks of cleansing or washing. They may be ashamed of wet or soiled underwear being seen, and prefer not to seek or accept help, even when needed. Where a carer and parent are of the opposite sex, considerable reluctance is common, and many middle-aged people do not wish to see their parents naked. It should never be assumed that because a relative is willing to care, he will also be at ease with all the tasks that this entails. A daughter who will readily feed, wash, and generally care for an elderly parent may draw the line at cleaning up excreta.

It should never be forgotten just how disruptive incontinence can be in the home, and a carer who will tolerate much inconvenience and hard work may find incontinence is the straw which breaks the camel's back.

Certain treatments for incontinence may be impossible to implement if no one is available to help. Bladder training can be particularly difficult. It is no use working out ideal toileting times for someone who is dependent and alone. No amount of medication or training can postpone micturition indefinitely. For the forgetful, an alarm clock may be useful, but it must be responded to appropriately and then re-set for the next time interval after use. Many people who are forgetful about toilet visits will not reliably re-set an alarm. There is a need for a 24-hour alarm system, capable of being pre-set at variable intervals (e.g. by the nurse), with no need for the patient to re-set it. The hard-of-hearing might benefit from a vibrating or visual alarm system; no such system exists at present.

This is not to suggest that bladder training is impossible for the disabled or forgetful at home (Rooney, 1982). Many people have devised systems to enable continence, whether involving neighbours or ingenious home-made devices.

Where the family is caring for a very incontinent person in the home, their role is crucial. Often the official support that is provided could be improved upon. Too often those who appear to be coping well are left alone, when really they could benefit from more help, both as support and practical measures. Sometimes voluntary bodies fulfil this role better than official agencies (e.g. Multiple Sclerosis Society, Spinal Injuries Association and other locally-run schemes), filling a gap and supplying education which ideally the National Health Service should provide. Much more could be done to ensure that care at home continues, and possibly to enable even more people to be looked after at home. The development of relatives' support groups, and more relief or holiday places to give regular rests, would do much to mitigate the burden.

The home environment

The home surroundings may present problems for two reasons – either because incontinence is spoiling the home, or because the surroundings are not conducive to continence.

Most people are house-proud, at least to some extent. There can be little doubt that uncontrolled incontinence can ruin any home. Soiling of chairs, carpets and beds, with the associated smell, can render a home unpleasant very quickly. Unlike institutions, few homes are planned with ease of cleaning in mind. Many fabrics, items of furniture and carpets are very difficult or expensive to clean, and some may be impossible to rid of a lingering odour. Waterproof covers for cushions and the mattress may help, but few people want to live on plastic chairs and linoleum. The embarrassment of a visitor inadvertently sitting on a wet chair may be great. Odour is often very apparent and difficult to eradicate. It is lessened by prompt cleaning-up after incontinence and by keeping soiled pads and linen in airtight containers. Proprietary deodorants may help (e.g. Ozium (Downs) and Atmocol (Thackray) sprays or Vaportek environmental deodorant (Franklin)).

Some homes make continence difficult for the elderly or disabled. The lavatory may be inaccessible because of location or size. Ideally there should be a lavatory on each level in a house, but this is seldom the case. Many modifications can be made and grants may be available to help with the cost (see Chapter 9).

Official and voluntary services

Districts vary, but many services may be available to help those who are incontinent at home. In practice, people are most likely to get services if they also have another disability, or if they have been hospitalised at some point. Those who gradually become incontinent in their own homes are much less likely to seek or receive assistance.

The district nurse will be a key person in assessing the individual's needs and in mobilising resources or referring for further help. The general practitioner should likewise be involved, but some are not motivated or interested and see incontinence as a nursing problem. Community nursing services are able to provide nursing care and advice, a bathing service for those with difficulties in personal hygiene, and in some instances an evening or night service if necessary.

The health visitor or geriatric visitor can advise the patient or relatives and teach methods of management or suggest sources of help. Any of these nurses may be responsible for ordering aids for the incontinent, depending on local policies.

Also involved may be the social worker to advise on grants for home modification and financial assistance. The community physiotherapist may help mobility and advise on correct lifting and transferring techniques. The community occupational therapist can assess self-care skills and improve these with instruction or aids. The chiropodist or optician may help a person to cope independently by improving walking and vision. The home help is often crucial in assisting the individual and maintaining his home. Some District Health Authorities have a delivery service for pads (although people are often expected to collect their own, or the district nurse has to deliver). Many Districts could improve upon their aids service, both in the range and quantity available and in delivery arrangements (see Chapter 13).

Luncheon clubs, day centres, or good-neighbour schemes can all provide the individual with people to help him to be continent or deal with incontinence. This potential can be enhanced by good training on incontinence for staff. However, some centres will not take incontinent people. Keeping up the incontinent person's motivation and outside interests is vital in promoting continence. People need a reason to make the effort to be dry, and if they have no outside contacts, apathy easily sets in.

Voluntary bodies may provide practical help and emotional support. The British Red Cross Society may provide nursing care or lend commodes. The Women's Royal Voluntary Service may provide visitors or clothing replacements. Many self-help groups for individual illnesses or disabilities act as powerful pressure-groups locally in demanding better services, as well as providing help to their members.

Laundry

Most incontinent people can, with a good appliance or pad, minimise additional laundry. A few of those with severe incontinence and not in receipt of good aids suffer a considerable burden of extra washing. Nurses in hospital, where soiled items disappear in a skip or down a chute and reappear as if by magic in a linen cupboard, often give little thought to how a frail person with limited amenities can manage at home. Even one change of clothing or sheets per day can be a problem. If it is happening many times each day the volume of laundry can be vast (Dobson, 1974).

Many incontinent people do not have good laundry facilities. A lucky few have a washing machine, spin dryer, and even a tumble drier. Some do not have even a decent-sized sink, hot water, or a garden for drying. In some cases the home is literally taken over by the volume of soiled or drying linen. If only one sink is available, it is unhygienic to have to wash soiled laundry in the same place as food and crockery. Arthritic hands cannot wring linen effectively, and the weak may not be able to wash efficiently, to remove all trace of soiling, so that infection risks and smell may result.

Large quantities of clothes and sheets are needed if washing is not to become an almost continuous task. Linen has its useful life shortened by repeated laundering. Replacement costs money and may be impossible on a fixed income or pension. Hot water, washing powder and electricity or laundrette costs can also be a burden.

It is unclear who is responsible for helping those who cannot manage their own laundry because of incontinence. Much legislation is permissive rather than directive, the boundary between the health and social services is uncertain, and arrangements are at local discretion. Most home helps will do the laundry, although some object, understandably, if linen is heavily soiled or offensive. But the home help will be as hampered as the patient by poor domestic facilities, and some laundrettes will ban those suspected of bringing in soiled items. Many do use laundrette facilities but this is far from ideal.

Some health or local authorities provide an incontinent laundry service. This is by no means available everywhere, and where there is a laundry there is often a waiting-list. Unless the service is very efficient and reliable the incontinent person is at risk of being left without linen when delivery is delayed. A few have collections and deliveries up to three times a week. Most are on a weekly basis, and soiled linen can become most unpleasant within that time. Some laundries are run in conjunction with a linen loan, which is essential where services are infrequent, because otherwise no one would have enough linen.

A few people can take advantage of facilities such as a laundrette at a day centre. Some local authorities will lend incontinent people a washing machine via the social services department. The nurse needs to find out which services are available locally to ensure those in need can benefit.

Families with handicapped children can apply for a grant to buy a washing machine and/or a tumble dryer from the Family Fund. People in receipt of supplementary benefit may be entitled to claim a single payment to meet extra costs incurred because of incontinence, for example to replace worn-out clothes or bedding. Additional laundry may also be paid for. For details of benefits, see Allbeson and Douglas (1984), *National Welfare Benefits Handbook*. Various voluntary bodies may also give help with clothing and bedding (e.g. Age Concern, Red Cross, St John Ambulance).

It is likely that as the use of good-quality disposables increases and supply problems are overcome (see Chapter 13), the burden of laundry will be relieved, enabling many more of those severely affected by incontinence to remain in their own homes, rather than going into institutional care.

Disposal

Where large numbers of pads are used, disposal can be a problem because of the sheer volume involved. Some people still have an open fire and can burn pads (except in smokeless zones), and others have a regular bonfire. Most people simply wrap pads in newspaper or a polythene bag and put them in the dustbin, which can easily be filled within a week. The legality of this practice is uncertain and it may contravene Public Health regulations in some areas. Refuse-collectors in many districts are not obliged to collect rubbish which is known to contain incontinence pads. In practice, most turn a blind eye, provided that a bin-liner is used. For smaller pads, sandwich bags, which are cheap and come with twist seals, are convenient. Larger pads can be put, several at a time, in pedal-bin-liners. An additional dustbin may be required.

Those who live in high-rise flats with communal rubbish chutes can experience problems. Bags may break open; domestic animals scavenging in the rubbish skips can distribute used incontinence pads over public areas, leading to embarrassing questions as to where they came from.

Some health authorities issue disposal sacks with their deliveries of incontinence pads. These may be heavy-duty plastic bags or waxed paper sacks. The Environmental Health Department may run a soiled-pads collection service on a weekly or more frequent basis. Indeed, some specify that all incontinence items should be collected by this service rather than by the domestic refuse service. However, such a service is not always popular, as a certain stigma is attached to those seen by neighbours to be using it.

Disposal is even more of a problem for the incontinent who venture out of the home. Few male public lavatories have any disposal facilities, and even female lavatories with sanitary-towel incinerators or bins seldom have a receptacle for larger pads. When visiting friends or relatives, it may be awkward to have to dispose of pads. If staying away from home for several days it often becomes impossible to disguise the problem. Many incontinent people, whether out for the day or at work, simply have to wrap up their soiled pads and take them home. This necessitates taking a large bag everywhere, and they may worry that an odour will be detected. Certainly lavatories for the disabled should have reasonably sized disposal bins for pads (although not all do). But the able-bodied cannot use these facilities without risking public disapproval.

With careful assessment of individual needs and good planning of services and resources, most incontinent people can be cared for in the community. Indeed, some of those who are currently in institutional care might be enabled to live at home if services were improved. The nurse's aim must be to ensure that the incontinent do not have their lives dominated by their condition and do not lose their independence because of it.

RESIDENTIAL AND HOSPITAL CARE

Institutions vary greatly in their approaches to incontinence, and it is difficult to generalise. Some offer excellent management and are geared to the promotion of continence; others are less imaginative and allow their residents minimal opportunity to become or remain continent. A few common problems are outlined here.

ACUTE CARE

Much incontinence occurs in acute, rather than long-stay, settings. It often starts on an acute ward and is the reason for eventual transfer to long-stay care rather than return to the community.

In acute hospitals, priority is given to the care of life-threatening conditions, and dressings, intravenous infusions and the administration of injections will usually take precedence over toileting. With the increased use of patient allocation and problem-orientated nursing care, it is now easier to identify priorities for each individual. Maintenance of continence needs to be given a much higher priority than it often gets at present. Most people would much prefer to be taken to the toilet promptly when they ask, than to have their bed made or lunch served on time. Nurses must learn to identify those of their patients 'at risk' of becoming incontinent in hospital – e.g.

immobile, confused, or depressed patients and those on high-dose diuretics – and take appropriate preventive action. If incontinence does occur, the nurse must find out why and plan care around treating it. Often the patient will be more disabled in the long term, not by the cause of hospital admission (e.g. a fractured neck of femur), but by the fact that incontinence was allowed to develop while in hospital.

There is a great temptation to use a catheter to manage incontinence in an acute setting – to protect a wound, minimise infection, or monitor urine output. This should be resisted unless there is a genuine need for a catheter (see Chapter 15). Patients are too often sent home with their catheter still in situ, or suffer catheter-related problems when it is removed.

When a patient is in hospital for rehabilitation, the success or failure of the rehabilitation programme will often be determined by whether his incontinence can be brought under control, either by cure or appropriate containment. All members of the rehabilitation team should be involved in trying to restore the individual to continence: the nurse in planning bladder training and creating a positive environment, possibly involving reality orientation or behaviour modification (see Chapter 8); the physiotherapist by mobilising the patient; the occupational therapist by improving dexterity and assessing which aids would be the most appropriate; the social worker by arranging any necessary adaptations to the home; and the doctor by the appropriate use of medication or specialised investigation. Continence is everyone's responsibility, but it will usually be the nurse who co-ordinates these efforts.

LONG-STAY CARE

Environment

Some residential homes and hospitals are purpose-built for the needs of the elderly or disabled. Good design can make continence easier, with plenty of accessible lavatories within a short distance of beds and day rooms. Floors should be non-slip and easy to clean, grab-rails plentiful, and corridors well lit with clear signs. Chairs and beds should be designed for ease of rising. The lavatory should be warm, clean and private.

Unfortunately, even some purpose-built accommodation does not fulfil all these criteria; and many homes and hospitals are not purpose-built, but are adapted from older buildings originally designed for a very different purpose. Hospitals for the elderly may be adapted from the old workhouse or fever hospitals, with Nightingale-style wards and minimal sanitary arrangements. Nurses are often far too good at coping and 'making do' in unsatisfactory environments. Both Wells (1980) and Reid (1974) have found that nurses tend to be uncritical of the toileting and changing facilities provided, being more likely to adopt ad hoc local routines rather than complaining or finding out how the situation might be improved. Residential homes may have been converted from large private houses with narrow corridors and numerous flights of stairs. This is not to say that such houses cannot be adapted successfully, but a great deal of thought, planning and usually money must be put into them if the adaptation is successfully to cater for the needs of the incontinent (see Chapter 9).

It is possible that too clinical an environment may encourage incontinence, especially in the confused. It has been observed that if the institutional setting closely resembles a normal 'home' environment, incontinence levels drop. Indeed, moving a group of long-stay patients from a hospital ward to a nursing-home environment, with more home comforts and an emphasis on reality orientation and personal responsibility, can dramatically reduce incontinence levels (Storrs, 1982).

Much can be done to transform an unsatisfactory environment. Nurses should get involved in planning, especially of new wards and homes, and demand necessary alterations where conditions are poor. It is too easy to put up with things and make do. In the long run this benefits nobody.

Staff

Institutions involved in the long-term care of incontinent people often have staffing problems. There is no doubt that the work may be heavy and unpleasant and can easily become a never-ending routine of changing, washing, and cleaning up, day after day. It may be difficult to attract staff, especially of a high calibre, and even more difficult to keep them. Staff turnover and sickness rates are often high and morale very low. Staffing levels may fall well below even the numbers funded. In some hospitals it is seen as a punishment or sign of disfavour to be allocated to a ward with high levels of incontinence. In both homes and hospitals there tends to be a high proportion of untrained or unqualified staff who, never having had any teaching about incontinence, tend to accept it as inevitable.

Staff attitudes are an important factor in incontinence. Even trained staff often have minimal knowledge about incontinence (Wells, 1980). It is easy, once working with incontinent people, to get so engrossed in the never-ending tasks of cleaning up that the reason for the basic problem is never questioned. It becomes accepted as inevitable. Once accepted, it is possible that residents are never given a chance to be continent. Routines become geared to mopping up rather than promoting continence (Ramsbottom, 1980). It is not uncommon for management methods to make it impossible for the individual to be anything but incontinent. Once privacy and dignity are lost, incontinence often becomes the norm.

Nobody likes cleaning up after incontinence. It is easy to see why staff develop routines which attempt to make incontinence easier to cope with. Doing a round with a trolley of dry pads and clothes and changing everyone in turn gets the job over with quickly and efficiently. By cutting off emotionally it becomes a task like any other, if you do not spend too long thinking about it. It is possible to argue that staff who have received no training on incontinence have no alternative to accepting such mindless rituals, and must, to tolerate the job, prevent themselves seeing or admitting what they are doing to other human beings. To change people in a communal room, in public view and while making infantilising comments, must mean that the staff are dissociated from the reality that they are dealing with another adult with a right to dignity. The old, the demented, and the disabled are too often dehumanised on account of their incontinence. The nurse must always strive to devise methods of care which, firstly, maximise the potential for continence and, if this fails, manage incontinence with dignity. The first step towards achieving this humane approach is to change staff attitudes towards incontinence.

The resident
Why do people who were continent at home start wetting soon after admission to an institution? The reason may be simply the physical cause for admission, such as a stroke, or immobility or other disease. Sometimes the change of environment may be the cause: taken away from their usual surroundings and methods of coping, they may be too shy or embarrassed to ask for the necessary help or to mention that they always keep a commode by the bed at night. Disorientation, or not knowing the proper words to ask for facilities, may lead to incontinence. They may find the staff threatening or unhelpful, and become unwilling to ask for the help they need.

If the admission is for permanent care, it is not unusual for a person to become depressed. This may be mistaken for 'settling down' and becoming adapted to the routine. The resident who sits quietly in a chair and makes no demands may make life easy for staff, but the fact that depression is the reason is often missed. Apathy may soon follow depression and incontinence may result. Why bother, if everyone else is incontinent and it seems to be expected? With the loss of independence in all the tasks of daily life some people regress to the point where everything has to be done for them; they cannot take responsibility for any aspect of life, including excretion.

Other factors may add to the problem. Lack of stimulus to keep active can lead to immobility. Arthritic joints seize up, independent walking becomes impossible. It therefore takes longer to get to the lavatory and help is needed. The immobile often become constipated, which in turn will aggravate urinary or faecal incontinence. Immobility may also aggravate fluid stasis in the lower limbs, which may then be treated with diuretics.

Once incontinence becomes established the sufferer, along with those around him, often assumes that nothing can be done and accepts it as inevitable.

Individual assessment

The importance of individual assessment of the patient or resident in long-stay care cannot be over-emphasised. Many studies have found that multiple problems are usually contributing to incontinence for each person, but that each will have a unique combination of factors needing attention (e.g. Lepine et al., 1979; King, 1979, 1980). Untreated medical conditions, drug side-effects, constipation, urinary tract infection, immobility, depression, disorientation, and a whole variety of other problems may be implicated (see Chapters 2 and 3 for the causes and assessment of incontinence). Until it has been discovered why each person is incontinent, any attempt at remedy is unlikely to be effective. Although such individual assessment is initially time-consuming, the long-term benefits are great, both in terms of the patient's dignity, and a more rewarding nursing workload.

TOILETING ROUTINES IN INSTITUTIONAL CARE

It is common for long-stay institutions to develop very rigid toileting and/or changing routines. This will usually involve toileting or changing (usually both) all residents at set times. This may be before or after meals and refreshments, or at a time which fits conveniently into the general routine. Such practices often go on year after year, regardless of whether they have any beneficial effect. Usually no record or chart is kept and the mindless routine is never changed.

This obviously does not fit with individualised patient care or a therapeutic regime. Although residents of institutions lead very regular lives, with regular fluid intake and activities, and so are likely to need toilet facilities at predictable times each day, these times will be different for each individual. One person may always need to pass urine half an hour after a cup of tea, but another may need to go two hours later. Trying to toilet everyone at the same time means that some will not need to go, while for others it will be too late. It also creates problems if insufficient lavatories are available, placing pressure on staff. Where task allocation persists it is often an unfortunate junior who is assigned the task of toileting a large number of people in a short space of time and having them all ready for lunch. Under such circumstances people are bound to feel hurried (and thus often inhibited from bladder emptying), and privacy is difficult with a queue outside.

In many places all incontinent people are treated identically by putting them on a toileting programme. Often this involves taking them to the toilet at pre-set intervals (every two to four hours). It has the advantage of being easy to remember, so that staff find it simple to comply. It will also keep a proportion of people dry by emptying their bladders before they really need to. However, it does nothing to diagnose the cause of the incontinence, nor does it retrain the bladder or the patient. Rigid regimes such as these are best reserved for those people, usually only the very demented, for whom all efforts at retraining have failed and whose incontinence is intractable. It will seldom apply to all those in one location. If a rigid regime is used, a chart should be kept to monitor the success of the chosen time-interval.

Certainly, in the first instance, the aim will be to retrain the bladder rather than merely to contain the incontinence. For a retraining programme toileting times will have to suit the individual's needs. (Chapter 4 above describes bladder-training for the mentally alert. Care of the elderly mentally impaired is dealt with in Chapter 8.)

The success of bladder training will depend on correct patient selection and diagnosis. It is pointless trying to 're-train' someone with stress or overflow incontinence; no amount of toileting is likely to keep them dry. It is most suitable for the mentally alert with urgency and frequency, and for the mildly to moderately confused with unpredictable incontinence. If the incontinence of a dependent patient is caused by a poor environment and low staffing levels, it is more often necessary to 're-train' staff to respond to the individual's needs and recognise their most suitable toileting times, than to train the patient's bladder. Offering toilet facilities at the times they are needed should be seen as part of basic nursing care and as a right for all patients. The term 'training' is more properly used to describe an effort to change those times and increase independence.

Much of what has been said in the rest of this book applies equally to people at home or in an institution, so this chapter should not be read in isolation. It attempts to highlight some of the more common problems associated with location of the individual. In practice many settings have been well designed, and those caring for the incontinent are doing all they can to promote continence and manage incontinence. Many excellent programmes, services, and facilities are in existence. Knowledge and resources need to be spread more widely so that this good practice can become the norm.

REFERENCES AND FURTHER READING

Age Concern and Disabled Living Foundation, 1979. *Improving Services for the Incontinent Adult; Report of a Survey.* Age Concern (England), Mitcham, Surrey.

Allbeson, J., Douglas, J., 1984. *National Welfare Benefits Handbook* (13th edn.). Child Poverty Action Group, London.

Browne, B., 1978. *Management for Continence.* Age Concern (England), Mitcham, Surrey.

Dobson, P., 1974. *Management of Incontinence in the Home – a Survey.* Disabled Living Foundation, London.

King, M. R., 1979. 'A study on incontinence in a psychiatric hospital'. *Nursing Times*, 75, 1133–1135.

King, M. R., 1980. 'Treatment of incontinence'. *Nursing Times*, 76, 1006–1010.

Lepine, A., Renault, R. K., Stewart, I. D., 1979. 'The incidence and management of incontinence in a home for the elderly'. *Health and Social Services Journal*, 89, E9–12.

Muir Gray, J. A., 1980. 'Incontinence in the community'. In: Mandelstam, D., (ed.), *Incontinence and its Management.* Croom Helm, Beckenham.

Ramsbottom, F. J., 1980. *Toileting and Changing Elderly Patients in Hospital.* Department of Geriatric Medicine, University of Birmingham.

Reid, E. A., 1974. *Incontinence and Nursing Practice.* M.Phil. thesis, University of Edinburgh.

Rooney, V., 1982. 'A question of habit'. *Nursing Mirror*, 154, 19, Community Forum ii-iv.

Storrs, A., 1980. 'What is care?' *British Journal of Geriatric Nursing*, 4, 12–14.

Wells, T. J., 1980. *Problems in Geriatric Nursing Care.* Churchill Livingstone, Edinburgh and London.

Chapter 12

Toilet-training the Mentally Handicapped

The majority of people with mental handicap, whatever their degree of impairment, have the potential to attain some degree of continence. In most cases, incontinence represents a failure to learn the skills necessary for continence. With others it may be related to behaviour problems. In both cases it should never be accepted as inevitable until a serious attempt at toilet-training has been made.

Some people suffer a co-existent mental and physical handicap and may have a neurogenic bladder problem as well. In such cases it is always advisable to investigate bladder function prior to initiating a training programme, as the training will not be effective if there is a severe underlying bladder dysfunction. Likewise, if the individual is so physically disabled that independence and self-help are precluded, any programme will have to be modified accordingly. The particular problems of the disabled and the neurogenic bladder are discussed, respectively, in Chapters 9 and 10 above.

Incontinence can be one of the most socially restricting aspects of mental handicap. Many otherwise feasible activities may be precluded because of it. If the person lives with his family, incontinence often forms one of the major burdens of care, in that the home may be physically spoilt, social activities restricted, and, not least, the physical burden of laundry, especially for the older child or adult, may be overwhelming. Considerable extra financial costs are common, as a Disabled Living Foundation survey has highlighted (Bradshaw, 1978), and this includes the costs of laundry, replacing clothing and bedding worn out by excessive washing, buying pads and equipment, and new furniture and carpets. As the individual grows, so also may the problem, until it can become the reason for breakdown of family care (or indeed breakdown of the parent's own relationship) and for requests for temporary or permanent care away from home. In recognition of this burden, the Family Fund (see Appendix of Useful Addresses) has resources to supply needy families with washing machines and other practical support not available from the statutory services.

If the mentally handicapped person requires a home away from the family, incontinence may be the deciding factor in placement. Many community-based residential hostels will not accept the severely incontinent. Those with self-help skills that are adequate in all other respects for some degree of independent living may be forced to live in a hospital because of incontinence. Current policy aims at considerably reducing the number of hospital beds for the mentally handicapped, particularly long-stay beds, and placing as many people as possible in community settings. This means that attaining continence has become one of the most important aims in rehabilitation. It should be noted that some people who have been doubly incontinent while in hospital care become continent when moved to a more domesticated environment in a community setting.

Hospitals which provide long-term care for the mentally handicapped often have the highest levels of incontinence encountered anywhere. Reports that nearly all individuals on particular wards or units are doubly incontinent are not unknown (Brown, 1972), and many patients have at least some degree of incontinence.

Wherever people with mental handicap live, incontinence is likely to cause considerable problems. Thankfully this is not inevitable, and it is increasingly realised just how much can be done in all settings. In the community, many District Health Authorities now have, or are setting up, community mental handicap teams to support clients either in their own homes or in residential accommodation. In hospitals, attitudes are changing from providing custodial care to more positive therapeutic interventions with the aim of maximising each individual's potential, whether to enable eventual community residence or to improve their quality of life in hospital.

As with most skills, teaching the mentally handicapped person to be continent is more likely to be successful the earlier it can be started. The ideal time to start training is probably around the second birthday, the age at which most non-handicapped children are toilet-trained. (Some training can start as early as 15–18 months, for example getting the child used to sitting on the potty.) This will usually be part of a larger programme aimed at achieving maximum independence in skills of daily living. However, if training has not been started early, this by no means indicates that the chance has been lost, and very high success rates can be achieved with older children, adolescents and adults who have either missed out or failed with training earlier in life.

Toilet-training the mentally handicapped is not a simple or easy procedure. It should never be started lightly, without consideration of the full implications. All those connected with the individual's care must be enthusiastic and willing to co-operate and work hard together as a team. Ideally the programme should be supervised by a professional trained in working with the mentally handicapped (nurse, psychologist, or other), usually with additional experience in using behaviour modification and operant conditioning techniques. The Registered Nurse for the Mentally Handicapped (RNMH) receives extensive instruction in such techniques during training, and the popularity of additional courses is increasing. Without such support, whether in hospital or community, any toilet-training programme will be more difficult to implement and will stand less chance of success. It is probably wise for those inexperienced in these methods not to attempt a programme without support and supervision, because the additional work and effort involved can rapidly lead to frustration and disillusionment with failures.

TRAINING METHODS

The ideal aim of toilet-training is independent toileting and continence. This may not be realistic for all individuals. Certainly there are so many elements involved that it is usually best to break down the skills required into a series of intermediate target steps or behaviours, which can be worked on separately or in combination. One method of dividing the steps, devised by Tierney, is shown in Table 12.1. The ultimate goal is to achieve the top final target behaviour in all four columns. Progress is indicated by ascending any of the columns from the base target behaviour, via intermediate targets, towards the final target. The end point may have to be accepted short of the top in one or more of the goals, depending upon a realistic assessment of the individual's physical and mental potentials.

Most programmes are based on the theories of behaviour modification. The underlying principle is that behaviours which result in pleasant consequences are thereby 'reinforced', and will tend to continue and become an established element of the individual's behaviour repertoire. Behaviours which result in neutral or adverse consequences are not reinforced and tend to be discontinued or

Table 12.1: Model for Shaping Toilet Behaviour

Final target behaviour	Patient goes to the toilet independently	Patient removes his clothing independently	Patient sits down on the toilet independently	Patient eliminates only in the toilet and is otherwise continent
Intermediate target behaviour	Patient asks to go to the toilet	Patient removes or actively attempts to remove some of his clothing	Patient is helped to sit down on the toilet and sits unrestrained	Patient eliminates in the toilet regularly and has only infrequent episodes of incontinence
	Patient indicates his need to eliminate	Patient actively assists when clothing is removed by nurse	Patient is placed on the toilet and sits unrestrained	Patient has established some regularity and uses toilet more frequently than is incontinent
Base target	Patient is taken to toilet by nurse	Patient co-operates passively when clothing is removed by nurse	Patient is placed on toilet and is restrained to sit	Patient uses toilet when placed on it but is incontinent at all other times

Tierney, 1973, reproduced by courtesy of the Editor, *Nursing Times* 'extinguished'. By close observation and careful planning, a programme is worked out to shape the desired behaviour gradually by the use of appropriate rewarding until a carefully defined target behaviour is attained.

Many different training methods have been used with mentally handicapped people, and most achieve a reasonable degree of success. The programme must be acceptable to and understood by those who will carry it out, whether family or staff. The main differences between approaches are in the timing of toileting, the use of reinforcers, and in residential settings, whether people are trained individually or in groups. Probably the most successful method is individualised intensive training using regular time-interval potting and mild correction for incontinence (Smith, 1979). Whichever method is chosen, the most crucial factor in success will be a consistent approach to training, i.e. having everyone who is involved with the individual approaching the training in an identical manner throughout the training period.

Intensive individual training involves a great commitment on the part of the trainer and may be very time-consuming during the initial stages. A method outlined and found successful in hospital by Smith is shown in Table 12.2. This method used regular potting, timed by the clock rather than to coincide with any pre-charted likely times for incontinence. This regular-interval training has usually been found to be simpler to carry out than toileting based on the individual's own natural bladder functioning.

The use of punishment in training is a controversial issue. Certainly many earlier studies, especially in the USA, used punishment or 'over-correction' to eliminate undesired behaviours. Today this is usually seen as unethical, especially the use of physical punishment. It has also been found to be largely unnecessary, and indeed may be counter-productive if it produces a high level of anxiety, since learning is impeded. However, a reprimand, or 'time out' from reward or attention for a specified time interval, are a commonly-used response to avoidable mistakes. This is probably helpful if given consistently and promptly. Some training methods also require the individual to participate in rectifying the consequences of incontinence (i.e. changing the bed or clothes), and this has in some instances been found to hasten learning (Barker, 1979).

Individual training is naturally used in the home. In residential settings a choice must be made between individual and group training. The former is much costlier in staff time than the latter, where one staff member may deal with a small group of patients. However,

Table 12.2:   General Guidelines for Regular Potting, Intensive Training

1) Bladder/training procedure	Seat child close to toilet Prompt to toilet every half-hour Reinforce (i.e. reward) for using toilet Reinforce every 5 minutes for dry pants
2) Accident/training procedure	Immediate and sharp reprimand when wet Feel wet pants for discrimination learning Do *not* change wet pants immediately Do *not* prompt to toilet 'Time out from reward' for 10 minutes
3) Independence/training procedure	Fade prompts to toilet, physical → verbal → gestural (in this order) Stop prompts when self-initiated toiletings established Move gradually away from toilet

Reprinted with permission from *Behaviour Research and Therapy*, **17**, 1, Smith, P., 1979, Pergamon Press.

individual training on a one-to-one basis usually takes less time to achieve continence and also tends to yield better results, so may be cost-effective overall. If staffing levels are such that it is impossible to contemplate individual training, then training a small group (say five or six) less intensively is a reasonable substitute.

BASELINE OBSERVATION

All toilet-training programmes should start with a baseline observation period. This will involve regular checks at pre-determined intervals to ascertain whether the individual is wet or dry, and careful recording of the results. Close observation should be made of episodes of incontinence as well as of the preceding and consequent behaviour of both the client and his carers. Families or staff may have developed styles of coping with and reacting to incontinence that can actually be eliciting the behaviour. The most common mistake is to give a lot of attention and create a lot of activity when incontinence occurs, and to virtually ignore the client when he is dry or performing continently. It is not difficult to see how this situation arises. Incontinence is experienced as a nuisance since, if not dealt with promptly, it can soil the environment and lead to smell. It is a natural reaction to hurry the incontinent person off to the bathroom to clean up the mess. While washing and changing the patient, most people will give him at least some attention and contact, both physical and verbal. Even if the content of the verbal exchange is a rebuke it constitutes attention, and some mentally handicapped people tend to respond to any form of attention as if to a reward. The incontinence is actually being rewarded. Conversely, dryness is seldom rewarded so consistently. When observing this behaviour pattern in carers it is important not to apportion blame to parents or staff, who are probably very caring, but to tactfully point out that this kindness may be counter-productive, suggesting how the attention might be reversed to reward continence rather than incontinence.

Observation of the client will indicate whether any warning is given of imminent micturition. Many will have no verbal skills, so this will usually be non-verbal, such as general agitation, getting up, or repetitive actions. Does the individual seem to be able to discriminate when he is wet? This might again be by agitation or wandering or by pulling at clothing or crying. Is he ever toileted, and if so, is urine passed appropriately? How many other para-toilet skills does he already have? Being able to walk, put on and remove clothing, sit upright unaided, wash hands, communicate simple needs verbally or non-verbally, and follow simple commands are all useful although not essential. Sometimes specially adapted clothing can improve the potential for self-care.

During this baseline period it is also important to establish what constitutes a reward for each individual. To an even greater extent than with the non-mentally handicapped, this group are not capable of conceptualising a distant, albeit worthwhile reward once the goal has been achieved. Something must be found which acts as a reinforcement to behaviour and which can be delivered immediately, simply, reliably, and frequently. This may be verbal – saying 'Well done', or giving a cheer. More often, non-verbal rewards may be better understood and appreciated. This might be anything from a smile or pulling a funny face to clapping, a pat, a hug or a kiss. The reward may be a drink or a sweet or other food. Care should be taken with edible rewards as the calories involved can lead to a weight problem and increase tooth decay. Likewise, fluid intake may already be excessive (which will exacerbate incontinence) because it has been found by carers that drinks act as pacifiers. This will not be harmful during training, since the greater the fluid intake, the more training opportunities will occur, but excessive frequency once trained will be undesirable. Also, if drinks are used as a reward during training, they should be strictly reserved for the relevant purpose and not given at indiscriminate times as well. Sometimes the reward can be linked to the toilet itself, e.g. using a musical toilet alarm or setting up an apparatus which will produce a noise when urine is passed onto it (Headingly Scientific Services).

It can never be merely assumed that something will act as a reward unless it has been proved that the individual will respond to it in some way. If the reward selected is actually disliked, or seen as neutral, it will not reinforce the desired behaviour. A noise might be found frightening, for example, or a selected food disliked. Often a small reward such as a sweet which can be easily kept in the trainer's pocket and delivered immediately is the best choice. The effectiveness of rewards should be reviewed regularly, as the desire for a given reward may reach satiation point, so that it becomes ineffective. If this occurs, new rewards should be introduced.

To be selected as suitable for toilet-training, the individual should be able to hold urine for at least one hour on some occasions and respond to simple rewards, and there should be someone, either a relative or a professional, prepared to carry out the programme.

THE TRAINING PROGRAMME

Most training programmes will take several weeks, and in some cases several months, to be effective. It is essential to keep accurate records throughout so that progress can be monitored and any necessary adjustments made (Woods and Guest, 1980). Records will also provide feedback to help keep up the motivation of all involved. This is probably the most crucial factor in success – that the programme is rigidly and consistently adhered to and not abandoned too soon. The community mental handicap team has a very important supportive role in the home, and although not always able actually to carry out the training, should be freely available for advice and encouragement to help maintain motivation.

Once any target behaviour is achieved, prompts should gradually be withdrawn (i.e. from actually escorting the client to the lavatory, to verbal and then gestural prompts), so that the behaviour becomes increasingly spontaneous and independent. This process is called 'fading'. Rewards should also change from being continuous (a reward for every correct achievement) to intermittent, with gradually decreasing frequency of reward (termed 'changes in reinforcement schedule').

Eventually the comfort and independence afforded by continence become reward enough in themselves to maintain the behaviour for some individuals. Others will need intermittent reinforcement and reminders to maintain continence after the programme itself is over. Some will never achieve total continence and will always need some help and reminders.

In a hospital setting, the introduction of toilet-training where it has never been used before often involves a considerable change in attitudes, and particularly re-thinking of nursing roles. This cannot be imposed from above or outside, as the staff must actively want to participate. At first it is often seen as a lot of extra work, and pessimism about the outcome is common. It is usually best to introduce the idea by means of staff training sessions such as study days and seminars, and start toilet-training in those areas where staff express an interest or request a programme. Likewise, it is a good idea to select patients for training whom the staff feel are appropriate and have a chance of attaining continence, certainly in the first instance. Pointing out the potential long-term benefits of reducing the proportion of time spent in toilet-related activities, and a more satisfying workload, may help gain enthusiasm for the project. All the staff on a ward, including ancillary and domestic personnel, must understand the training, so that consistent responses are shown by all members of the care team.

Some mentally handicapped people exhibit other behavioural problems in addition to incontinence. It has often been found that these improve during a toilet-training programme. General levels of self-help skills and independence are also often increased as an additional benefit. This is probably a result of the increased attention and stimulation offered within the learning environment afforded by toilet-training.

Sometimes using a pants alarm (see Figure 5.2) or toilet bowl alarm (Figure 12.1) help greatly during the training. These enable carers to know immediately when incontinence or micturition has occurred and to take the appropriate action promptly. The more closely the consequence is paired with the act, the stronger will be the conditioning effect. However, care should be taken that the individual does not respond paradoxically to alarms; i.e. a few may enjoy the pants alarm and wet intentionally to create the noise, or alternatively be frightened by the toilet alarm and withhold urine on the toilet.

Nocturnal enuresis may be corrected by similar, but obviously less intensive, behaviour modification programmes. Dry beds should be

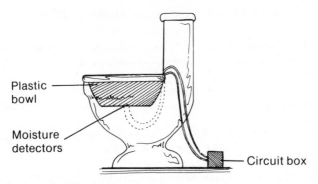

Figure 12.1 *Toilet-bowl alarm.*

rewarded and regular potting encouraged at pre-determined intervals. Probably encouraging participation in changing wet beds will aid learning. Alternatively, the enuresis alarm can be effective if well supervised (see Chapter 5), and used as part of a wider behaviour modification programme.

CONTAINMENT

A minority of mentally handicapped people are unresponsive to toilet-training. Others live in situations, either at home or in hospital, where training is not feasible. For such people an efficient method of containment is of paramount importance, and often very difficult. Some may not tolerate appliances, and even pads and pants tend to be pulled at or removed. The problem of containment is especially great when the client is an adult, who may empty a full bladder with considerable force. There is as yet no adequate answer for this and some clients are obliged to remain in institutional care on account of it.

It may be that the 'diaper' all-in-one systems (see Chapter 13) or extra-large terry nappies are the best available at present for most mentally handicapped adults with total incontinence. However, these tend to be expensive and many health authorities are reluctant to provide them. A very good case of special need and priority often has to be made to procure a supply, but there can be little doubt that if the provision of an expensive pad enables the individual to be cared for at home, this is a good use of resources, on both humanitarian and financial grounds.

REFERENCES AND FURTHER READING

Azrin, N. H., Foxx, R. M., 1971. 'A rapid method of toilet-training the institutionalised retarded'. *Journal of Applied Behaviour Analysis*, 4, 289–299.

Barker, P., 1979. 'Nocturnal enuresis: an experimental study involving two behavioural approaches'. *International Journal of Nursing Studies*, 16, 319–327.

Bradshaw, J., 1978. *Incontinence, a Burden for Families with Handicapped Children.* Disabled Living Foundation, London.

Brown, J., 1972. 'Ward 99'. *Nursing Times*, 68, 7, 197–201.

Sines, D., 1983. 'Incontinence: helping people with mental handicap'. *Nursing Times*, 79, 33, 52–55.

Smith, P. S., Britton, P. G., Johnson, M., Thomas, D. A., 1975. 'Problems involved in toilet-training profoundly mentally handicapped adults'. *Behaviour Research and Therapy*, 13, 301–307.

Smith, P. S., 1979. 'A comparison of different methods of toilet-training the mentally handicapped'. *Behaviour Research Therapy*, 17, 1, 33–43.

Tierney, A. J., 1973. 'Toilet-training'. *Nursing Times*, 69, 1740–1745.

Tierney, A. J., 1980. 'Toilet-training the mentally handicapped'. *Nursing*, 1, 18, 795–797.

Woods, P. A., Guest, E. M., 1980. 'Toilet-training the severely retarded; the importance of evaluation'. *Nursing Times Occasional Papers*, 76, 18, 53–56.

Chapter 13

The Use of Incontinence Aids

There is a a huge range of aids and equipment produced to help incontinent people. These aids aim to preserve the individual's dignity and self-respect by making it possible to conceal and manage the incontinence. By containing urine or faeces the aid should enable the person to feel and be socially acceptable again.

In the past the provision of aids has all too often been seen as the be-all and end-all of incontinence management. The nurse has assessed the incontinent patient with the selection of the most suitable pad or appliance paramount in her thoughts. This outdated practice has to a great extent been superseded by a more positive, problem-solving approach. However, even with the best available nursing and medical care, not all incontinent people can be completely cured. There is always likely to remain a sizeable minority whose problem persists despite all efforts. There will also be those who are too ill for therapy, or who make an informed decision not to undergo recommended treatment. Some may be improved considerably but still wish to use an aid to give them confidence in public, and many will need a temporary supply while awaiting or undergoing treatment.

SELECTION OF INCONTINENCE AIDS

People require and expect many different things from an aid. The ideal aid should fulfil the following criteria. It should:

(a) be fail-safe, i.e. contain the excreta completely and prevent any leakage through to clothing or the environment at any time and under any circumstances.

(b) be comfortable to wear and protect vulnerable skin from soreness, chafing or pressure sores.

(c) be easy for the incontinent person to use and manage for themselves. Where this is not feasible due to physical or mental disability, it should be easy for the carer to use.

219

(d) disguise or contain any odour.

(e) be easily concealed under clothing, neither bulky nor noisy, and so be inconspicuous in use.

(f) be easy either to dispose of, or wash and clean, as appropriate.

(g) be reasonably priced and easily available.

Some people will also have their own particular requirements, such as being reasonably attractive so as to fit their personal body image, or easy to pack and transport for travellers. Some like disposable items, others prefer to wash and re-use an aid. This list could be extended almost indefinitely. Each incontinent person's priorities will be unique to him as an individual.

There is considerable confusion over the proliferation of incontinence aids. The most comprehensive catalogue is produced by The Association of Continence Advisors (*ACA Directory of Aids 1984*). This lists the personal aids available in the UK and the main source of supply for each (over four hundred different aids with a hundred different companies). It is beyond the scope of the catalogue to offer detailed recommendations on selection, and only brief advice is given on the uses of generic types of aids. The Disabled Living Foundation produces a leaflet for use by professionals or the public which lists examples of most types of aid, but again offers only minimal advice on detailed selection.

Historically, many items produced for use by incontinent people have been poorly designed, with little thought put into the real needs of the user. Often pads have been conceived merely as larger versions of babies' nappies, without realising that the needs of an ambulant adult are likely to be very different. Many appliances were very heavy and cumbersome, with multiple straps, belts, and connections which were difficult to use and provided many potential weak spots for equipment failure. Today considerably more thought is going into product design, and modern science and technology are employed for the benefit of the sufferer. Many companies have realised that there is a potentially vast market for incontinence products, particularly if those who at present hide their problem can be persuaded to come forward and seek help (see prevalence of incontinence figures, Chapter 1).

It is only very recently that substantial investment has been devoted to new product development, and many of the benefits of this are yet to come. Many of the items described in this chapter represent the results of the first wave of interest, and are likely to be rapidly superseded over the next few years as the returns from this investment in research become apparent.

There are many reasons why companies have taken so long to recognise the potential market presented by incontinence. Incontinent people are difficult to identify as a market. If they do not seek professional help they cannot be supplied with aids via the National Health Service, and these same people are also likely to be too embarrassed to purchase their own aids. Those who do use aids are often so grateful for any help that they are uncritical of what is provided. Their expectations are often very low, and few complain if an item is inefficient – almost anything compares favourably with nothing. Nurses and others caring for the incontinent have tended passively to accept whatever was supplied, being unaware of alternatives. Few have been vocal in demanding the best for their patients. The National Health Service has failed to stimulate interest in developing high-quality products, because contracts have generally been awarded with price as the primary consideration. Manufacturers have almost been forced to produce to a price, rather than to a quality, and as a result there are many poor-quality, and some frankly shoddy, items being sold. There is little incentive to develop high-quality products if these do not sell. With increased professional interest and public discussion about incontinence, companies are at last seeing a future for quality products. It is now realistic for them to market a product on the basis of its particular merits rather than produce bedpads or penile sheaths similar to those of other companies.

A big problem, when recommending aids, is the lack both of convincing clinical trials and technical quality-control tests for almost all items. The International Standards Organisation and British Standards Institution have now set up committees to draft technical standards for aids for ostomy and incontinence. The results of their deliberations are awaited with great interest. Most aids do not have even one published trial evaluating their use. Nearly all trials have been very small-scale, with a few notable exceptions (e.g. Malone-Lee et al., 1983), and almost none comparative. There is therefore very little basis on which to make a choice other than personal experience. It is impossible to tell how an aid will perform without trying it – some items that look and feel to be of high quality have a design fault which stops them fitting, whereas other very unlikely-looking aids may be the perfect solution for someone.

There is some reluctance to try new aids. If the present supply is 'good enough', then newer items, with possibly superior qualities, may be ignored. Both users and professionals tend to have very low expectations of performance – all too often it is expected and accepted that the aid will be uncomfortable and smelly, and leak from time to time. Nobody enjoys having to wear an aid, but if one must, it should not be necessary to expect such a poor performance.

SUPPLY OF AIDS

The supply of incontinence aids is not always straightforward or easy. Fewest problems are encountered in the community with collection devices such as catheters, bags and male appliances, as most are available on prescription by the general practitioner. The Drug Tariff (Part 1XA) lists all items available on prescription and gives guidance on the usual expected life of the aid. However, most general practitioners have no specific training and still find selection from the many items difficult, especially if there is no fitting service available. The selection of a specific product may be left to the retail pharmacist, who may be equally lacking in knowledge or training. Some pharmacists deal with only one wholesaler, who may not stock the exact item requested and will provide a substitute. Others have difficulty in obtaining small quantities, and will only order and stock certain sizes or types. The provision of an appliance on prescription, without a fitting service or follow-up supervision of its use, cannot be ideal for the patient. Perhaps community nursing services should increase their involvement in this with a view to improving patient care.

In the UK, with the exception of Scotland, the health authority takes responsibility for the supply of absorbent aids to the patient in the community, usually via the district nursing services, although sometimes jointly with the social services department, and occasionally via the social services department alone. In Scotland, bedpads (but not body-worn pads) may be obtained on the GP's prescription, provided that they meet specifications laid down by the DHSS (London).

In general, regulations about what should be made available to the patient are permissive rather than directive. Contracts are often awarded Regionally, and each Authority is encouraged to purchase within the contract. With little evidence except price to go on when awarding contracts, it is not uncommon for the contract to be awarded to the contender whose price is the lowest, regardless of quality. Supplies Committees cannot be blamed for such decisions if they are not receiving good advice from clinical personnel, and few clinical nurses make it their business to track down the people who make these decisions, to influence them for the good of their patients.

Individual health authorities vary greatly in what they are prepared to provide for incontinent people. Most have certain 'stock' items that are reasonably easily available. Some hold a reasonable selection of absorbent aids from which it should be possible to meet most needs; others provide a bare minimum (e.g. only bedpads). Some authorities will only buy from within the Regional contract; others are prepared to negotiate separately if they feel their needs cannot be met from within the contract. The difference between health authorities, even those immediately adjacent geographically, can be quite startling, and there is a great inequality of provision of absorbent aids across the country. Most authorities do have a 'special order' system whereby an item that is not kept in stock may be obtained by a special requisition. Usually this is authorised by a senior nurse manager. In practice this system functions badly in many instances, and in some areas it is impossible to obtain items to suit individual requirements. Many community nurses are unsure what their, or their patients', rights are in relation to the provision of aids, and merely accept the stock item regardless of individual needs. 'We cannot get it' is, in practice, more often a case of 'We don't know whom or how to ask for it'.

Supply problems in hospital likewise depend on local circumstances. Some hospitals insist on buying in bulk, and so will only order a single pad for all needs. Others will allow ward sisters or senior nurses to be more flexible and order a range of items.

In view of the fact that a good reliable aid can make such a difference to the life and well-being of an incontinent person, those areas where supply is problematic warrant investigation and appropriate remedy. Naturally there are many competing needs for money in the National Health Service, but it should not be beyond the realms of feasibility to devise a system by which a selection of thoroughly tried and tested aids is available free of charge to anyone who has need of them. Possibly the UK could learn from Sweden in this respect. There, all community nurses have a catalogue of 'approved' and tested aids which they can prescribe for their patients. These prescriptions are processed centrally and then sent to a distribution centre, for direct delivery to the patient. It is likely that a similar system could operate in the UK. However, it is unlikely that retail chemists could cope with this as they lack both storage space and delivery facilities, so the health service needs to look at its own supplies system. Not only could the quality of the incontinent person's life be improved, but in the long term such a system could also be cost-effective, enabling patients to stay in the community and live independent lives rather than possibly needing institutional care.

In practice, most incontinent people currently buy their own aids. For those who can afford to do so, or have minimal leakage, this matters little. However, some people who can ill afford it are forced to purchase their own aids, either because they will not seek professional help, or because National Health Service provision is inadequate in quality or quantity. It is not uncommon to meet an incontinent elderly woman who is 'rationed' to so many pads per week, but who really needs twice as many and has to make up the balance from her own pocket. Usually this means buying sanitary towels or baby diapers from a chemist, which can be very expensive, especially to someone on a pension or low income. Some will buy by mail order, from newspaper advertisements. A few seek personal help from commercial appliance-fitters or showrooms. Some people prefer to buy aids privately, but for the majority it represents a financial burden, coupled with the fact that they often receive no advice or help on selection or suitability; and if obtained by mail order, no fitting or guarantee of performance. There is also a tendency for those who can disguise their incontinence to delay indefinitely the point at which they pluck up the courage to seek professional help.

ASSESSMENT

The key to the success or failure of an aid will usually lie in an accurate initial assessment of the patient's needs. There is no one aid that will suit everyone. The nurse must make an assessment, with the range and uses of the available aids in mind, so that a decision can be made with the patient and his carers (if relevant) as to the item most suited to his needs. It should never be forgotten that a patient's needs may change with time, so the assessment of suitability must be a continuing process, and supply systems flexible enough to accommodate changes. Nurses must challenge policies such as 'All incontinent people get one box of pads per fortnight' as being unlikely to meet the needs of any but a few individuals.

When making an assessment for the provision of aids, the following points will be of particular significance.

The incontinence itself, including type (urinary or faecal); amount (how much is lost in total volume); pattern (is this a single flood, occasional large amounts, frequent small amounts, or a continuous dribble); precipitants of incontinence (e.g. is it stress, urge, or passive incontinence); timing (night only, only when out, only after diuretics, only when suffering bronchitis). Also of note are other urinary symptoms, such as frequency and urgency.

Mobility. The bed-bound, chair-bound and ambulant patient have different needs. The sportsman or woman will have different requirements from an aid from someone who leads a more sedentary life.

Manual dexterity. If dexterity is poor some aids cannot be managed easily or independently. For example, particular disabilities may determine the particular type of outlet tap that can be used.

Local anatomy. Features of the genital skin condition or anatomy may indicate or preclude certain items. Of particular note are a retracted penis, hernias or scrotal swellings, skin sensitivities or lesions, obesity, and any particular deformities.

Mental function. A confused or demented person will seldom be able to manage a complex aid unless help is available. Some will not even be able to put on a pad correctly, if at all. If the patient denies any problem of incontinence, it will usually be fruitless giving them an aid, as it will not be used.

Personal hygiene. People vary greatly in their levels of hygiene. The fastidious may use an aid differently or require a different aid from someone with poor hygiene. Washable and re-usable aids are often inappropriate for those unlikely to wash them properly.

Personal preference and perception of need. Some people take a like or dislike to certain products. For example, some men dislike the idea of pads. The look and feel of a product may influence choice, and some people will refuse to try something just because of the way it looks or because they do not like the idea of it. These personal preferences should be respected wherever possible; it is, after all, the patient who has to wear and rely on the aid.

Official services. The availability of help from the district nurse, home help, laundry or disposal services may influence management.

Availability. An easily and reliably available aid may be preferable to a more suitable but unreliably or intermittently available one where there are supply problems. However, this situation should not be allowed to continue indefinitely, and the nurse should make every effort to get the most suitable aid reliably supplied.

Domestic facilities available for washing, drying or disposal.

Regular help. For those with impaired mental or physical function, some aids will only be usable if someone else is regularly available to help.

Financial considerations. The NHS has to be cost-conscious, and cost must be a factor if several items are genuinely equally suitable. Additional equipment which might be necessary in order to use certain aids, such as a washing machine, might also be precluded because of cost.

It cannot be emphasised too often that aids will seldom be the first line or only management for incontinence. Nobody's problem may be assumed intractable until fully investigated. The majority are curable.

The remainder of this chapter outlines broad types of aids, mentioning currently available examples. Addresses of suppliers/ manufacturers are given in Appendix 1.

When supplying any aid it is essential to teach the patient and carers how to use it correctly, including application, removal, cleansing or disposal. The nurse should also check periodically that the aid is being used appropriately (written instructions may be useful for the forgetful). A suitable aid will be ineffective if it is used wrongly, and it is surprising how many patients will use even the simplest aid inappropriately (for example, applying a pad with the plastic backing next to the skin). Regular re-evaluation of the use of the aid should ensure both that the patient's needs have not changed and that a newer, more suitable aid is not now available.

PADS AND PANTS

The use of an absorbent pad worn inside a retaining garment is the most common way of managing incontinence. For women, there is no satisfactory external collection appliance and pads are the only way of collecting leakage. Many men, especially those with a retracted penis or poor manual dexterity, also use pads, although some feel that pads are 'feminine' and prefer to use an appliance if at all possible.

A considerable amount of technology lies behind the design of a good incontinence pad, and much thought has been put into the manufacture of the better products. However, there are also many low-quality products in existence, often using cheap materials such as reprocessed newspaper instead of virgin wood pulp. Unfortunately it is extremely difficult to spot inferior products until they are in use, when their performance is usually poor. It is very important to ask the manufacturer what a pad is made from and to try it in practice, before making large purchasing decisions. At present, there is no central quality control of pads in the UK.

The most readily available and most commonly used pad is a sanitary towel. If a brand with a plastic backing is used it will cope successfully with minimal leakage. The advantages of using a sanitary towel are that it is small and unobtrusive under clothing, reasonably comfortable, easily available, and easy to dispose of in a public lavatory. They are 'normal' for women to wear, so may not make the user feel conspicuous as 'incontinent'. The disadvantages are that, for greater than minimal leakage, several of them may have to be worn at a time; if a brand without plastic backing is used, urine tends to leak straight through onto clothing; the cost can be considerable; and many elderly women feel embarrassed buying them. For those with slight or occasional incontinence who can afford sanitary towels, they are the best solution. For anything heavier, a specially designed pad is usually more satisfactory.

Three broad categories of garments may be distinguished: an absorbent pad worn inside waterproof pants; plastic-backed pads worn inside a retaining garment; and all-in-one garments ('diaper' system).

Pads with waterproof pants
Plastic pants were for many years the only form of incontinence aid available. Many designs are simply large versions of babies' plastic pants made from polyvinylchloride (PVC) with elasticated legs and waist. Some have straps to retain the pad in position. Drop-front and side-opening varieties fastened with tapes or poppers are also available. Many people feel that plastic pants are very safe and would trust nothing else. They are also reasonably cheap. They do have many disadvantages in that they tend to be uncomfortable, hot and sticky, and rustle a lot. With repeated washing the 'plasticiser' which makes the PVC soft leaks out and the plastic soon becomes hard and brittle, with cracks developing. Plastic pants can be the cause of considerable skin damage and cause excessive perspiration. They are also so closely associated with babies and nappies that many adults find wearing them degrading. Their use cannot be recommended except in special circumstances (such as for the young patient with very healthy skin for

a limited period of time), and most patients who are using them can easily be weaned off them when they discover that the alternatives are just as safe and much more comfortable.

Attempts have been made to improve plastic pants. Some are made from heavy-duty plastic in order to prolong their life. This generally results in the pants being very stiff and even more noisy and uncomfortable. Others are lined with material to prevent direct skin contact with the plastic, which may reduce discomfort to some extent.

Many pants have a plastic gusset rather than being all plastic. This considerably reduces heat and discomfort. The Brevet 'Sanitas' pants (Figure 13.1) are made from a white lacy material and have adjustable side fastenings, elasticated waist and legs, and lined plastic in the crotch, extending well up at the front and back. Henley's 'Sandralux' pants (Figure 13.2) are a fairly standard pair of women's stretch pants with a smaller gusset of waterproofing stitched into the crotch. These are popular because of their resemblance to ordinary pants.

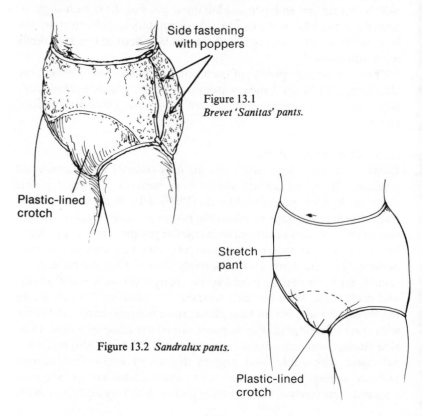

Side fastening with poppers

Figure 13.1
Brevet 'Sanitas' pants.

Plastic-lined crotch

Stretch pant

Figure 13.2 *Sandralux pants.*

Plastic-lined crotch

The 'marsupial' pants are an attempt to provide waterproof pants without having any plastic near the skin. Kanga Pants (Figure 13.3) were the first example of this, although now several other makes are available. They are made of a soft knitted hydrophobic material, elasticated at the waist and legs, with a waterproof pouch for the pad on the outside of the pants. Because the material is hydrophobic it does not absorb liquid into its own fabric. When urine is leaked it should pass through the pants into the pad in the pouch. So long as the pad is changed before it is soaked, the material next to the skin should stay dry, and urine be conveyed away from the patient's skin. In practice this is not totally effective as the material does hold some liquid, but this dries quickly with body heat. Marsupial pants are certainly popular, possibly because they were the first real alternative to all-plastic pants. They need to be fitted carefully, as a close fit, especially around the hips and legs (where the elastic is adjustable), is necessary to prevent leakage. They are unsuitable for use in bed, for faecal incontinence, and for patients with a vaginal discharge, as the pants become stained. Some people dislike the idea of wetting their pants directly and of keeping the soiled pants on after wetting. Fear that they will smell, and a feeling of remaining damp, are common. Many prefer to have a changeable pad next to the groin. Considerable dexterity is also needed to insert and remove the pad from the pouch. They have the advantage that they can be used as a normal pair of pants if the pad is placed in the pants before they are put on, which is often easier than holding a pad to the crotch and trying to pull a pair of pants up over it. Confused people who would not remember to

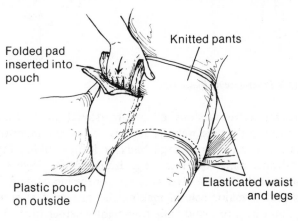

Figure 13.3 *Kanga pants.*

replace a pad can be allowed independent toileting in the knowledge that when they pull up their pants the pad will automatically be in place. Those who tend to pull at their pad and remove or destroy it may wear the pants back to front so that they cannot get at the opening of the pouch, which is then behind them. Women need the pad placed centrally in the pouch, men need it more towards the front. Marsupial pants are only suitable for those with reasonable levels of personal hygiene and who are able and likely to wash the pants thoroughly each day.

In addition to the standard marsupial pants, variations can also be obtained in a side-opening or drop-front design with Velcro and/or popper fastening. This enables the pants to be put on and taken off without being pulled over the legs. They are useful for those in wheelchairs or with calipers, and may help those using a hand-held urinal in a chair (Figure 13.4).

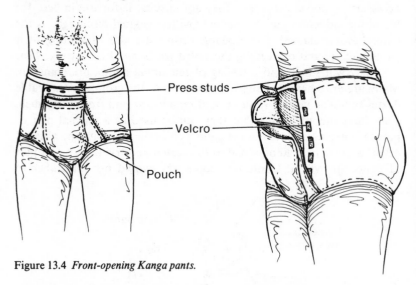

Figure 13.4 *Front-opening Kanga pants.*

More attractive versions of the marsupial pants enable many patients to feel they are wearing acceptable normal underwear. Pastel colours for women (e.g. Kanga Lady or Kanga Bikini, Figure 13.5) and 'Y-front' pants for men (e.g. Kanga Male, Figure 13.6) are popular. As self-image is often very low for the incontinent, ideas such as this play a major role in making the sufferer feel acceptable to society, and help to avoid embarrassment whether in the laundrette, changing-room, or with a partner.

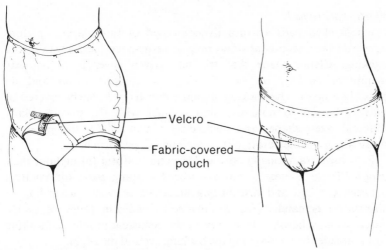

Velcro

Fabric-covered
pouch

Figure 13.5 *Kanga Lady and Kanga Bikini pants.*

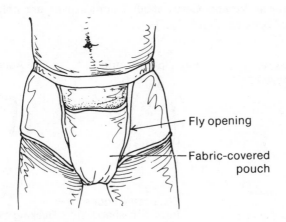

Fly opening

Fabric-covered
pouch

Figure 13.6 *Kanga Male pants.*

Pads which go inside waterproof garments have no waterproof backing themselves, and are therefore relatively cheap. Many different sizes and thicknesses are available and selection should be tailored to the patient's needs. Rolls of absorbent material which can be cut to any length have the advantage of flexibility for varying needs, but some patients cannot manage to cut a roll easily. Some rolls are of very poor quality and the absorbent material falls apart in use.

231

Plastic-backed pads

Plastic-backed pads are usually composed of three layers – a non-woven surface, absorbent wood-pulp or tissue-paper, and a waterproof backing. Claims made that the non-woven cover is a 'one-way membrane' to keep the skin dry have never been proven and are possibly a myth. The backing should either be completely covered or microembossed to minimise skin contact with the plastic. Many different sizes, shapes and thicknesses are available, and generally those which use the best-quality materials will perform best.

Pads have traditionally been oblong and uniform throughout their length. There is now a move towards shaping pads for comfort between the legs and distributing materials unevenly, according to absorption demands, (e.g. Mölnlycke's Tenaform range of pads). Attempts have been made to prevent the persistent problem of leaking from the sides by overlapping the backing around the edges.

For light incontinence, a sanitary towel is the smallest and most discreet pad. Several pads are designed to take volumes of 50–100ml. The Mölnlycke Tenette is shaped; the LIC Daisy pad is elasticated for a 'cup' effect; Vernon Carus small Cumfies pads are oblong with overlapped backing (Figure 13.7).

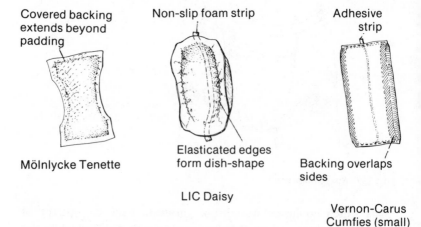

Covered backing extends beyond padding

Mölnlycke Tenette

Non-slip foam strip

Elasticated edges form dish-shape

LIC Daisy

Adhesive strip

Backing overlaps sides

Vernon-Carus Cumfies (small)

Figure 13.7 *Pads for light incontinence.*

For moderate incontinence, most pads are of the standard oblong design, e.g. Robinsons Inco Care Insert, Vernon Carus Medium Cumfies pad.

People leaking over 150–120ml into a pad need a large pad. These can be very bulky but are necessary to contain the leakage. They may be oblong (e.g. Mölnlycke Maxi-Plus pads, Ancilla inserts), shaped (e.g. Mölnlycke Tenaform Normal and Extra), or wing-folded (e.g. LIC Deolic, Ancilla Wing-folded pad) (Figure 13.8). These pads are all long, and patients with limited dexterity find it difficult to hold them in place while pulling up pants. Extra-large pads are available for night use (e.g. Mölnlycke Tenaform Super).

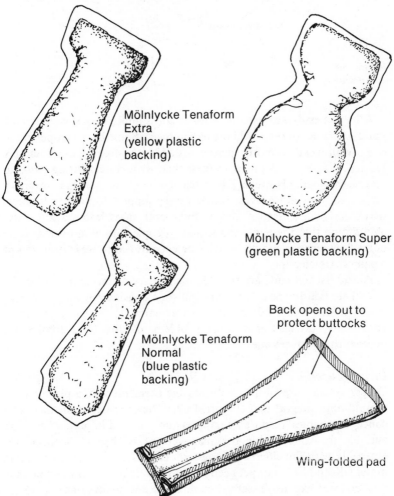

Mölnlycke Tenaform Extra (yellow plastic backing)

Mölnlycke Tenaform Super (green plastic backing)

Mölnlycke Tenaform Normal (blue plastic backing)

Back opens out to protect buttocks

Wing-folded pad

Figure 13.8 *Pads for heavy incontinence (see also overleaf).*

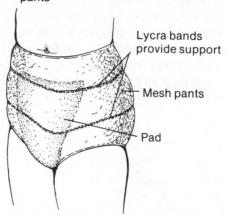

Mölnlycke TenaFix
pants

Lycra bands
provide support

Mesh pants

Pad

Figure 13.8
(continuation)

All these pads are usually worn inside simple, inexpensive stretch pants, designed only to hold the pad in place. Some have an open mesh (e.g. Mölnlycke TenaFix pants), others are slightly more closely knitted. Some people prefer to wear their own closely fitting pants to retain the pad. However, it must be emphasised that ordinary underwear may not provide the necessary support to prevent leakage, particularly in cases of heavy loss, and may lead to the false assumption that the pad is inadequate. People who wish to wear their normal underwear should perhaps be encouraged to wear it on top of a pair of stretch pants.

Plastic-backed pads are suitable for urinary or faecal incontinence. It is likely that the next few years will see a considerable improvement in the design and trials of alternative materials. The use of super-absorbents may also grow if the problems of slow fluid uptake and expense can be overcome.

Diaper systems

Diaper systems are all-in-one disposable garments with a plastic wrap around and integral pad (Figure 13.9). They are based on the same concept as babies' disposable nappies and are used in parts of Europe and North America for the management of heavy incontinence, especially with the elderly in long-term care. They are not as popular in the UK and have not yet been properly evaluated. It is possible that this relatively expensive method could be acceptable in some situations, especially if versions with elasticated legs, self-adhesive patches, and a non-woven material lining the plastic are used. However, many patients react unfavourably to the association with babies, and they do tend to rustle and be rather hot.

The use of pads and pants may present problems with washing the pants. If so, the light mesh pants are usually easiest to wash, although they do not stand up well to hospital laundries. Disposal of pads can also be problematic if incontinence is heavy (see pages 200–201).

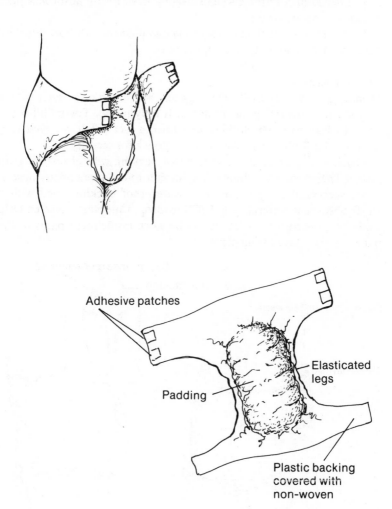

Figure 13.9 *All-in-one diaper.*

MALE APPLIANCES

The male anatomy offers greater potential for the successful use of appliances than does that of the female. The penis can be inserted into a collection device or have an appliance attached to it, thus avoiding the distribution of urine over the entire perineum. Men with faecal incontinence or a retracted penis usually have to use absorbent pads rather than an appliance.

There are three distinct types of male appliances – dribble pouches, penile sheaths, and body-worn appliances.

Dribble pouches

Dribble pouches, as the name suggests, are suitable for men with a very slight or dribbling incontinence. It only takes a few millilitres of urine to leak through clothing and form a wet patch, so even very occasional dribblers may like to wear a pouch for security.

Pouches may be made of waterproof backing with absorbent pulp inside. These tend to be bulky and difficult to disguise under trousers. More successful are pouches with waterproof backing lined with a super-absorbent material (e.g. LIC Licodrop, Coloplast Conveen Drip Collector, Figure 13.10). These can be worn inside mesh pants or the patient's own close-fitting pants.

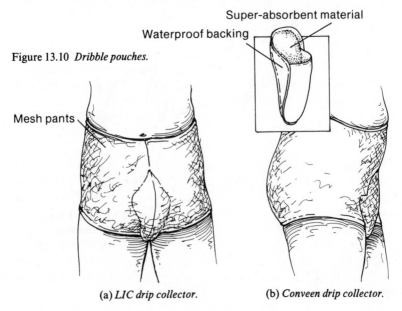

Figure 13.10 *Dribble pouches.*

(a) *LIC drip collector.*   (b) *Conveen drip collector.*

Washable dribble pouches may be worn on a waist-belt, jock-strap style. The pouch may be filled with wadding and changed as necessary (e.g. Downs Nupron Pouch, Figure 13.11).

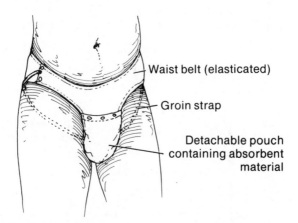

Figure 13.11 *Nupron dribble pouch.*

There are also some fairly crude dribble bags available, often just a plastic bag with a hole for the penis and possibly waist and leg tapes. These are not generally to be recommended.

Dribble pouches are not available on prescription.

Penile sheaths

A penile sheath is a soft, flexible, latex sleeve which fits over the penis and attaches to a urine-collection bag. It may also be referred to as a condom urinal, an incontinence sheath, or an external male catheter. Sheaths are designed to collect urine voided incontinently from the penis and store it in the bag until it can be conveniently emptied. A sheath is suitable for men suffering moderate to severe urinary incontinence, and may also be used for men with urgency or frequency in circumstances where it would be difficult to make repeated visits to the lavatory. It may be worn continuously or intermittently (e.g. just at night or when going out). Two types of sheath are available (Figure 13.12, overleaf). Type 1 is a very soft, thin, one-size latex sheath gathered distally into a rigid outlet tube. It may have a foam ring to cushion the tip of the penis. Type 2 is a thicker, less flexible sheath with a reinforced moulded distal end and outlet tube; it is available in a range of sizes from paediatric to extra-large.

237

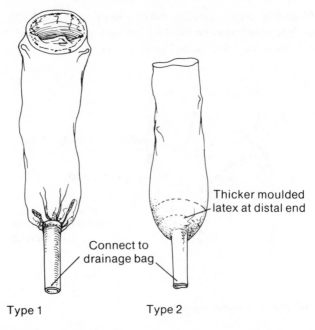

Type 1   Type 2

Figure 13.12 *Penile sheaths.* (a) *Type 1 (one size).* (b) *Type 2 (various sizes, from paediatric to extra large).*

Penile sheaths are not suitable for men with a very small or retracted penis, as attachment is impossible. Some men have a skin sensitivity to the latex and therefore cannot use sheaths. If the patient is to apply and manage his own sheath a reasonable degree of manual dexterity, good eyesight, and a fair mental capacity are needed. Demented or confused patients may repeatedly pull a sheath off and will almost certainly be unable to cope alone.

Some people use no method of attachment with a sheath, relying on having the correct size to hold it in place. Generally only non-ambulant patients can manage this, and most ambulant men need some method of holding the sheath in place. The simplest, but probably least effective, method is a strip of tape or adhesive foam wrapped around the outside of the sheath. Because no adhesive attaches to the skin the sheath easily slips off. Somewhat more effective is a foam-and-elastic re-usable band fastened with Velcro (e.g. Martin Creasey, Posey sheath-holder), but again there is no direct skin adhesion.

The most effective way of securing a sheath is by direct adhesion to the skin of the penis. This should never be done with ordinary surgical tape as it is not designed for the sensitive penile skin. Repeated application can cause skin problems, the incidence of skin sensitivities is high, and there is seldom enough elasticity in the tape to allow for erections. Three methods of skin adhesion are designed for use with sheaths. Double-sided adhesive foam strips tend not to have good elasticity and not to return well to their former length if stretched. Some tend to absorb urine and then to lose their adhesive qualities. Strips of 'Stomahesive'-type material are also adhesive on both sides, and can be applied around the penile circumference and the sheath then rolled up and over and pressed down to stick. Conveen Uriliner (Coloplast) is a very flexible version of this with a good 'memory', so that it returns to its original length after stretching and can be overlapped with safety. Medical adhesives probably give the most secure fixation of all. They may be spray-on (e.g. Dow Corning Medical Adhesive B), brush-on (e.g. Thackray Aquadry Medical Adhesive; Dow Corning Brushable Adhesive B), or in a tube of glue (e.g. Warne Medical Adhesive). The adhesive is applied around the circumference of the penis, allowed to dry for a few moments, and the sheath is then rolled over it and pressed down. The spray version tends to be difficult to direct accurately. Some men find the adhesive rather too adherent, and repeated removal may cause sore skin.

The selection of sheath and adhesive will depend on the patient's preferences and any known skin sensitivities. The sheath should always be large enough to fit easily over the penis and to allow for changes in penile size. Prior to applying the sheath the genital area should be washed and thoroughly dried. It is best to avoid using any creams or powders if adhesive is to be used. Long pubic hairs around the base of the penis should be trimmed short. If adhesive is used this should be applied about half-way along the shaft of the penis (Figure 13.13, overleaf), the sheath unrolled about 3cm and then, making sure the foreskin is not retracted, unrolled over the penis. It is important to leave a gap between the tip of the penis and the outlet tube to allow a small reservoir for sudden gushes of urine and to avoid pressure on the penis. If, however, this gap is too large the sheath may tend to twist, so that drainage is impossible. This is a particular problem with Type 1 sheaths.

If the sheath has a reinforced ring around the base of the penis, the ring may be cut to prevent pressure problems. The outlet tube is then connected to a suitable drainage bag. All bags used with indwelling catheters are suitable for use with sheaths, and selection will depend on assessment of the patient's needs and wishes (see Chapter 15).

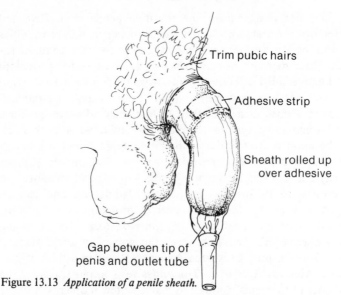

Trim pubic hairs

Adhesive strip

Sheath rolled up over adhesive

Gap between tip of penis and outlet tube

Figure 13.13 *Application of a penile sheath.*

When first applied as a new method of management, a penile sheath should be observed and checked regularly to look for any signs of constriction, skin sensitivities, or pressure. The sheath should be changed daily at first and the skin carefully inspected. Once the sheaths have proved satisfactory, each sheath can safely be left in place for one to three days between changes, depending on circumstances.

To remove the sheath applied with adhesive, simply roll both off together. The medical adhesives often have their own remover to take off any glue left behind. Simple soap and water will remove most. If adhesive is used, the sheath has to be disposed of and a new one used. If the sheath has not been stuck it may be washed, dried, and re-used. If the patient voids normally at times, it is usually best to disconnect the sheath from the bag rather than remove it completely each time.

Most penile sheaths, adhesive, and drainage bags are available on prescription in the community.

Body-worn appliances
There is a proliferation of male appliances, and many variations are available. All of these devices are expensive, and skilled fitting by an expert is essential. Many of the older models were very cumbersome, with multiple straps and connections, and were made of heavy rubber. The more modern versions are lighter and simpler, but there remains much scope for improvement, especially in comfort and ease of use.

Drip-type urinals are designed for men with light to moderate incontinence. They comprise an internal sheath and an external cone to collect urine, with waist and groin straps (Figure 13.14). An additional collection bag may be attached to give a greater capacity (e.g. Bard McGuire Urinal).

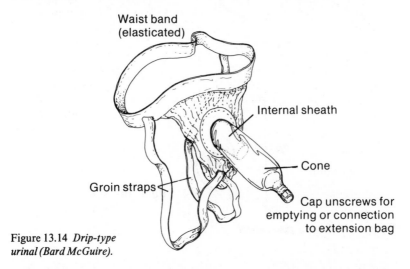

Figure 13.14 *Drip-type urinal (Bard McGuire).*

Pubic-pressure urinals have a semi-rigid pubic-pressure flange which is held closely to the pubis by waist and groin straps. This pressure may correct retraction and allow the penis to protrude into the urinal (e.g. Downs Pubic Pressure Urinal, Figure 13.15, overleaf).

Diaphragm urinals have a flexible diaphragm, held by straps through which the penis passes into the urinal (e.g. Thackray Adult Male Urinal, Figure 13.16, overleaf). Penis and scrotal urinals contain the whole genitalia and can be used with a severely retracted penis (Figure 13.17, overleaf).

Appliances come with many variable features. Some have an internal sheath to hold the penis and prevent backflow. Some have a scrotal support. Some are all rubber, others have material or elastic straps and plastic drainage bags. Bag capacity can range from 100–750ml. Some bags are free-hanging, others have leg-straps. Bags may be thigh-worn or used on the calf with an extension tube. Some are one size only and must be cut to fit the individual; others come in graduations of $\frac{1}{8}$ in. of penile circumference (measured next to the body with penis in flaccid state). Outlet taps, connections and straps may all vary and be easier for some patients than others.

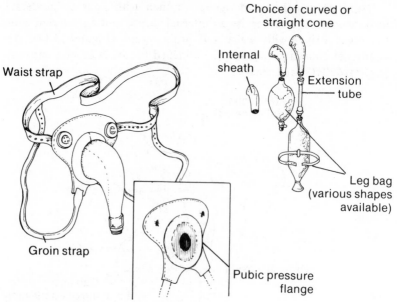

Figure 13.15 *Pubic-pressure urinal.*

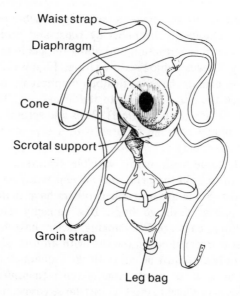

Figure 13.16 *Diaphragm urinal.*

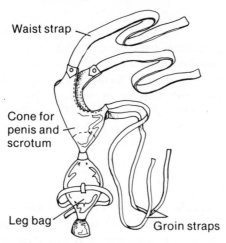

Figure 13.17 *Penis and scrotum urinal.*

The patient must have a reasonable level of personal hygiene and be willing to wash and clean the appliance regularly. Each patient will need two urinals – one in use and one being washed and dried. A mild antiseptic solution for cleaning may help to reduce any odour.

Many of the companies who make these devices have a specialised fitting service, and a nurse who is new to this field will usually do best to ask for their help or advice. Special items can often be made up individually if the patient has a particular problem. Most of these appliances are available on prescription.

BED PROTECTION

When a heavily incontinent person is wetting the bed some method of protecting the bed and skin will be needed (unless an appliance is being used).

Mattress covers
Various grades of waterproof mattress-cover are available to fit single or double beds. For long-term use the heavier-grade plastics are best. Elasticated edges make putting the cover on and keeping it in place easier. Many mattress covers are hot, uncomfortable and noisy. Covers should be wiped clean when changing bed linen to prevent odour occurring.

243

Draw-sheets

If urine loss is not too heavy a draw-sheet may be preferred to a full mattress-cover. Restless patients may find a draw-sheet is easily displaced. A draw-sheet may be a simple plastic sheet to be used under a linen washable draw-sheet, or a completely disposable sheet with an absorbent surface and waterproof backing (e.g. Mölnlycke Maxi Draw-Sheet; ACS Medical Draw-Sheet). These disposable sheets can be very useful for someone at home with washing difficulties.

Disposable underpads

Disposable underpads or bedpads are possibly one of the least effective and most misused of all the items that nurses use. The National Health Service consumes vast quantities (estimated over £7-million worth in 1982) and yet very little research has been done to study their effectiveness. The most commonly used pads are made from five layers of low-quality tissue-paper or wadding with a plastic backing. This type does not meet DHSS standards for absorbency and will not cope with anything but the smallest leak. Any sizeable leak results in the patient lying in a puddle, and very often the undersheet gets wet as well. The pad protects neither the patient nor the bed. Claims that one-way covers protect the skin are unfounded.

Thicker, better-quality underpads are available. Although more expensive, they are much more likely to protect the bed and possibly the patient (e.g. Smith and Nephew Polyweb bed-pad; Ancilla bed-pad).

Where underpads are used they should be laid across the bed with the sealed edges at top and bottom, so that if urine is going to leak out it will do so away from the patient rather than towards his head and feet. The commonly seen nursing practice of using several underpads on top of each other is both expensive and senseless. 'Packing' a patient at night – i.e. wrapping him in five or six underpads is costly and does little for the patient or bed. It is much more effective to use one good-quality pad than several cheap ones, and also usually cheaper in the long run.

Underpads should really only be used for faecal incontinence or slight urinary leakage in bed, or as a back-up in case a body-worn pad leaks in bed. Some health authorities will still only supply underpads and expect patients to cut them up to use inside pants in the daytime. This is no longer acceptable, and nurses must become more vocal in demanding better provisions.

Washable bed protection

The Kylie sheet (Nicholas Laboratories) is a washable draw-sheet for moderate to severe urinary incontinence in bed. It has a hydrophobic upper layer of pink polyester viscose, quilted to a lower layer of hydrophilic rayon. When urine comes into contact with the top layer it passes through rapidly without being absorbed into the substance and is soaked up and retained by the lower layer. The Kylie should be used on top of a plastic draw-sheet, and the cotton flaps tucked in either side of the bed (Figure 13.18). The incontinent person should lie directly on the sheet without nightclothes below the waist (a split-back nightdress or nightshirt may be useful). Urine is quickly dispersed and will not flow back and form a puddle, even under pressure, so the patient's skin remains relatively (although not absolutely) dry.

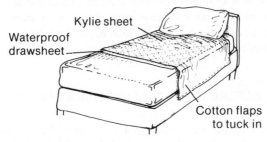

Figure 13.18 *Kylie bed sheet.*

Although the sheets are quite expensive, they have been shown in trials to be cost-effective if used correctly, saving money on laundry and disposables (Smith, 1979). They are also effective in preventing pressure sores for patients at risk of skin breakdown. Full co-operation from laundry services is vital if the Kylie is to be used in hospital. It is not suitable for faecal incontinence nor for those living at home without a washing machine and good drying facilities – because they hold fluid so well they can be difficult to dry. When saturated, the sheet is very heavy and cannot be managed by a frail person alone. A recent product launched on the market has a cotton facing, an integral waterproof backing, and is somewhat lighter (Dagonais sheet, ACS Medical).

A washable sheet is especially popular in residential homes and in the community, where washing facilities allow. If there is no helper on hand to change the incontinent person, and where he or she cannot manage alone, it can allow an undisturbed and comfortable night's sleep.

Body-worn pads

The use of body-worn pads rather than bed protection at night is gaining popularity. The larger plastic-backed pads (e.g. Mölnlycke Tenaform Super) or a diaper system (e.g. Peaudouce Slipad) may be used. It is possible that a pad which holds urine close to the body and thus keeps it warm will increase patient comfort and decrease disturbed nights. Much more extensive trials are necessary to evaluate the relative merits of protection of the bed and patient.

The huge amount of research and development of incontinence aids currently being undertaken means that many items described here will soon be obsolete. This is all to the good. Nurses should keep abreast of new developments and, indeed, encourage them by being willing to purchase the best available for their patients. Each patient who needs an aid is different, and the nurse must be able to assess individual needs accurately and know which aid is most likely to help to contain the problem of incontinence.

REFERENCES AND FURTHER READING

Association of Continence Advisors, 1984. *Directory of Aids* (second edn.).

Disabled Living Foundation, Incontinence Information Service, Notes No.12, London.

Malone-Lee, J., McCreery, M., Exton-Smith, A. N., 1983. *A Community Study of the Performance of Incontinence Garments.* Department of Health and Social Security, Aids Assessment Programme, London.

Smith, B., 1979. 'A dry bed – and save on costs'. *Nursing Mirror*, 148, 22, 26–29.

Chapter 14

Faecal Incontinence

If any problem is more embarrassing and less socially acceptable than urinary incontinence, it is incontinence of faeces. Whether in the home or in hospital, coping with faecal incontinence is a considerable burden and very unpleasant for both the sufferer and his carers.

As with urinary incontinence, faecal incontinence is a symptom which must have a cause. Accurate diagnosis of the underlying problem can lead to a very high cure-rate, and with good management, persistent uncontrolled faecal incontinence should be rare.

It is likely that about one adult in every two hundred living in the community suffers regular faecal incontinence. It tends to be a very under-reported symptom which many elderly or disabled people and those with ano-rectal disorders or diseases of the colon accept and disguise without seeking medical help (Leigh and Turnberg, 1982). However, by far the greatest proportion of faecal incontinence occurs in the elderly in long-stay institutional care. Many surveys of patients in geriatric or psychogeriatric hospitals have reported faecal incontinence in up to half of all patients, and certainly a prevalence of 10%–20% is common. On general hospital wards, 2%–3% of patients are likely to be incontinent of faeces (Egan et al., 1983). This high rate in hospitals adds enormously to the burden of nursing or caring for long-stay patients, and to the unpleasantness associated with the job. In the majority of cases it is a reversible or avoidable situation.

FAECAL CONTINENCE

Most people maintain faecal continence by virtue of a delicate co-ordination of the neurological and muscular activity of the colon, rectum and anus. The main function of the large intestine is to receive chyme from the small bowel, to absorb water from the chyme to form faeces, to correct some electrolyte imbalances, and to store and propel faeces. About 600ml of chyme are received per day, and this is eventually reduced to 150–200ml of faecal matter.

Movement of matter along the colon may be stimulated by physical activity, by neurological activity, by emotions, or by eating. Both eating and the sight or smell of appetising food cause the caecum to empty into the colon (the so-called gastro-colic response, which is probably mediated hormonally), and this often stimulates a 'mass movement' of faeces over great distances through the colon.

When faeces enter the rectum there is an immediate sensation of rectal fullness and impending defaecation. The sensory nerve endings responsible for this are probably located in the muscle around the rectum rather than the rectal wall itself. When the rectum is distended by about 150ml of faeces, the internal anal sphincter, which is a smooth-muscle (autonomic) sphincter, relaxes completely, allowing faeces to pass into the anal canal. The external sphincter, however, which is striated muscle, is under both autonomic and voluntary control (Figure 14.1). If defaecation is not convenient the external sphincter is contracted and the full defaecation reflex is inhibited from continuing to completion. The external sphincter maintains a continuous tonic contraction, even at rest, and this can be greatly augmented for short periods by voluntary contraction. If the defaecation reflex is voluntarily inhibited, the stool will be returned to the rectum until a

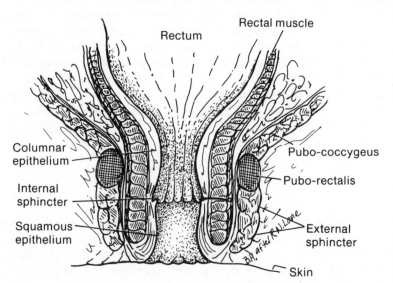

Figure 14.1 *Diagrammatic coronal section through the pelvic floor.*

more convenient time. The anal canal is lined with very sensitive squamous epithelium, which can distinguish accurately between gas, fluid and solid matter entering the anal canal, even during sleep. This is important as flatus can be passed without faecal incontinence occurring, and even fluid diarrhoea can be retained by most people.

If the defaecation reflex is not inhibited, i.e. if it is convenient to defaecate, the external sphincter will relax completely and with minimal abdominal effort rectal contractions will expel the stool, aided by gravity.

The muscular supports of the pelvic floor, especially the pubo-rectalis muscle, help to maintain a double right-angle between the anus and rectum which acts as a flap valve (Figure 14.2). This aids continence during physical activity. If abdominal pressure is raised, the pressure merely closes the valve more effectively. This is important in preventing stress incontinence of faeces. There is also a reflex contraction of the pelvic floor in immediate response to effort.

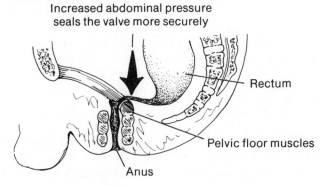

Figure 14.2 *The anatomical arrangement at the ano-rectal junction results in the formation of a flap valve. The anterior wall of the lower rectum impinges upon the closed anal canal and any increase in abdominal pressure seals the valve more securely.*

'Normal' bowel habit varies greatly between individuals. It is likely that 99% of adults in the UK have bowel motions between three times per day and once every three days (Connell et al., 1965). However, it should be remembered that what has become 'normal' on a highly refined Western diet is often far from optimal, as the high incidence of bowel disorders in the West testifies. One good-volume, formed, but soft and easily passed stool per day, without excessive urgency, flatus, or abdominal discomfort, is probably the best objective for most people to aim at. Variations upon one per day are seldom cause for concern unless these other criteria also fail to be met.

THE CAUSES OF FAECAL INCONTINENCE

Broadly, the causes of faecal incontinence can be divided into three categories: those indicating an underlying disorder of the colon, rectum or anus; neurogenic; and that resulting from faecal impaction.

UNDERLYING DISORDERS

Severe diarrhoea
Severe diarrhoea increases the likelihood of being faecally incontinent. Table 14.1 lists some of the more common disorders which can cause diarrhoea and faecal incontinence. The latter tends to be a common, if seldom reported, accompaniment.

Table 14.1: Common Causes of Diarrhoea

Ulcerative colitis
Crohn's disease
Villous papilloma of rectum
Carcinoma (may also cause constipation)
Infection
Radiation
Drug-induced (e.g. broad-spectrum antibiotics, laxative abuse, iron)

Those with impaired mobility, diminished sensation or awareness, or already impaired sphincter function are more at risk of diarrhoea causing incontinence than otherwise healthy individuals. Lower-bowel carcinoma is the commonest malignancy of old age, and any recent change in bowel habit should be thoroughly investigated in all age-groups. The remedy of this incontinence will obviously involve treating or bringing under control the underlying disease process.

Muscle-ring deficiency
The muscles of the pelvic floor support the anal sphincter, and any weakness will cause a tendency to faecal stress incontinence. Figure 14.3 shows that with muscle weakness the vital flap-valve formed by the ano-rectal angle is lost. Rises in abdominal pressure will therefore tend to force the rectal contents down and out. This may be the result of congenital abnormalities or of later trauma (e.g. obstetric, after anal surgery, or direct trauma such as in a road traffic accident). A

lifetime's habit of straining at stool may also be implicated in muscle weakness.

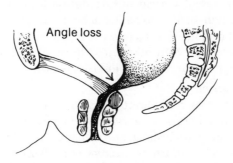

Figure 14.3 *With muscle weakness the flap valve formed by the ano-rectal angle is lost.*

Mild weakness may respond to pelvic-floor exercises. These should be taught very much as exercises for urinary stress incontinence (see Chapter 6) but concentrating on the posterior rather than anterior portion of the pelvic floor. Rectal tone should be assessed on digital examination and the patient instructed to squeeze. Regular contractions of the posterior portion of the pelvic floor should then be practised very often (usually five contractions per hour) for at least two months. The patient must also be instructed very firmly to desist from all straining during defaecation. Most people with muscle weakness severe enough to cause incontinence of solid stool require surgical repair to restore continence. The most successful surgery involves restoring the ano-rectal angle and flap-valve mechanism (Parks, 1980).

There is some evidence that straining or obstetric trauma may not only cause direct muscle damage but also damage the nerve supply of the pelvic floor by prolonged stretching of the nerve fibres (Parks, 1980). If the straining has also induced rectal prolapse this will require repair at the same time.

NEUROGENIC DISORDERS

The medulla and higher cortical centres of the brain have a role in co-ordinating and controlling the defaecation reflex. It is therefore likely that any neurological disorder which impairs the ability to appreciate or inhibit impending defaecation will result in a tendency to incontinence, similar in causation to the uninhibited or unstable bladder. For example, the paraplegic may lose all direct sensation of and voluntary control over bowel activity. Neurological disorders such as multiple sclerosis, cerebrovascular accident and diffuse dementia may affect sensation, inhibition, or a combination of both. Incontinence occurring in the demented person will sometimes be because of physical inability to inhibit defaecation. With others it is because the awareness that behaviour is inappropriate has been lost (see below).

The paraplegic patient
Often the patient does get indirect indications of when the rectum is full and defaecation imminent. Various autonomic indicators, such as tachycardia, sweating, or flushing, are often present and it is important for each individual to learn to become very sensitive to his own internal indicators if continence is to be achieved. If the lesion is above the cauda equina then it is usually possible to stimulate a defaecation reflex voluntarily, once the period of spinal shock is past. This is only useful if the rectum is full, so each person must learn to diagnose a full rectum correctly and then act upon it before an involuntary reflex causes incontinence. For many, the reflex can be initiated by dilating the anus, either with a finger or an anal dilator.

Cauda equina lesions
Where the defaecation reflex is disturbed because of damage to sacral nerve roots S_2 and S_3, defaecation is often extremely difficult to manage and total uncontrollable incontinence is common. The sphincters, devoid of nerve supply, are usually lax and patulous and simply allow faeces entering the rectum to pass straight out.

If a person with neurogenic faecal incontinence fails to achieve adequate voluntary control, the problem is best managed by artificially inducing constipation and then planning controlled bowel evacuations. Some authors recommend using a constipating agent in the morning (such as chalk and opium) and a laxative in the evening (e.g. senna preparations). Possibly a more reliable method is constipating the patient over several days and then emptying the bowel every three to five days with the aid of an enema or suppositories. Up to seven days will do little harm so long as no discomfort is experienced. A regime should be worked out to suit the needs, diet and life-style of each patient (Avery Jones and Godding, 1972).

FAECAL IMPACTION

Severe constipation with impaction of faeces is probably the commonest cause of faecal incontinence, and it certainly predominates as a cause among the elderly and those living in institutional care. Chronic constipation leads to impaction when the fluid content of the faeces is progressively absorbed by the colon, leaving hard, rounded rocks, or scybala, in the bowel. This hard matter promotes mucus production and bacterial activity, which causes a foul-smelling brown fluid to accumulate. If the rectum is overdistended for any length of time the internal and external anal sphincters become completely inhibited and relaxed, giving a completely patulous sphincter which freely allows passing of this mucus as 'spurious diarrhoea'. The patient's symptom will usually be of a fairly continuous leakage of fluid stool without any awareness or control. Obviously, if the diagnosis of the true cause of this is missed and the patient wrongly treated for diarrhoea with constipating agents, the condition will be aggravated. Some of the scybala may also be passed from time to time by gravity or pressure from the formation of more faeces above. Most patients with an impaction will have hard faeces in the rectum, but in a few the impaction is higher up and cannot be detected by digital examination.

The causes of constipation
Constipation, the underlying cause of faecal impaction with consequent faecal incontinence, has itself many possible causes (Table 14.2).

Table 14.2:   Common Causes of Constipation

Cause	Examples
Simple constipation	Low-residue diet Dehydration Environmental factors
Motility disorders	Irritable bowel syndrome Idiopathic megacolon
Psychiatric disorders	Depression Confusion Anorexia nervosa
Local pathology	Anal fissure Haemorrhoids (piles)
General pathology	Endocrine disorders (e.g. diabetes, hypothyroidism) Carcinoma
Iatrogenic	Drug-induced Immobility Nursing management

'Constipation' means different things to different people, and is a difficult term to define. In practice, frequency of defaecation matters little, so long as the motion is of a soft consistency and easy to pass without undue effort or straining. 'Constipation' refers to motions which are hard and difficult to pass, usually also at irregular or infrequent time intervals.

Simple constipation. Simple constipation, i.e. that with no underlying bowel pathology, is often self-induced. It may be caused by low food or fluid intake (low fluid intake often being caused by fear of urinary incontinence); poor diet, especially one low in fibre or residue (in the elderly this may be for financial reasons or because of inadequate teeth to tackle fibre); or lack of exercise. As seen earlier, physical activity is an important stimulus to colonic activity, and mass movements are rare in the immobile. Diminished awareness may lead to ignoring the call to stool.

The environment may be important in causing constipation. Many lavatories are too high to allow the feet to rest comfortably on the floor, so additional help from the abdominal muscles cannot be employed during defaecation. This may be especially important in the elderly, whose muscle tone may already be decreased. Lavatories which are cold, uncomfortable, or inconveniently situated may encourage both the ignoring of rectal sensations, and allowing inadequate time for a completed bowel action. Privacy is also important for complete defaecation, and where privacy is lacking defaecation may be delayed or only partial. This may be true of a child at school, inhibited by the older children having a secret cigarette in the lavatory, or by no locks on vandalised doors. It may be the person who shares accommodation and fears that others are waiting. Or it may be the patient in hospital who can hear the nurse hovering outside the door and waits until next time in the hope of less haste and greater privacy. Many people have the ability to delay defaecation almost indefinitely, and impaction may result.

Motility disorders. The normal transit time of food through the gastrointestinal tract has been measured by radio-opaque markers, and is between three and seven days from mouth to anus for most people. Disorders such as the irritable-bowel syndrome or diverticular disease (itself probably caused by the constipating effect of Western low-residue, low-fibre, high-carbohydrate diet) can lead to constipation, sometimes alternating with diarrhoea. Some people have an idiopathic slow transit time or megacolon, and it is likely that transit time increases with advancing age. Slow transit time (eight to fifteen days is not uncommon) through the colon allows increased water absorption and encourages the formation of impaction. In the elderly this may lead to the 'terminal reservoir syndrome' where a hugely distended lower colon is never completely emptied.

Psychiatric disorders. Of prime importance here is depression, which is an often neglected cause of constipation. Confusion and dementia also predispose an individual to constipation. Conversely, constipation may be the underlying cause of confusion. Anorexia nervosa, self-purgation and some of the psychoses may underlie apparent constipation.

Secondary to local or general pathology. A large-bowel carcinoma may present as constipation. Haemorrhoids, anal stricture, or any painful ano-rectal disorder will tend to cause inhibition of defaecation and thereby constipation. Endocrine disorders, notably hypothyroidism and diabetes, may be the underlying pathology.

Iatrogenic. Constipation may be drug-induced (analgesics, especially opiates, anticholinergics, and anti-Parkinsonian drugs are among the many having this effect), or may develop because of a period of enforced immobility (e.g. post-operatively). It may also be induced by nursing management: for instance, requiring a patient to defaecate perched on a bedpan in bed – a most unnatural act, both because of the inappropriate position adopted and the lack of privacy. The straining and effort, not to mention stress, involved in attempting defaecation on a bedpan are often considerably greater than the effort of getting up to use the commode or lavatory. In cardiac patients, straining at stool is a known precursor of cardiac arrest and sudden death.

Constipation in the elderly

An old person may have a combination of many of the above-mentioned problems causing constipation. Wilkins (1968) has described a vicious circle of constipation in the elderiy (Figure 14.4, overleaf) which shows how factors combine to maintain constipation.

Many elderly people are obsessed with their bowels, often from a lifetime's habit of weekly purgation and persistent beliefs that a bowel which is not completely cleared regularly can become toxic. The elderly often attribute any feeling of malaise or ill health to too infrequent bowel actions. Many are chronic laxative abusers (Connell et al., 1965). This practice in itself may cause problems and eventually damage colonic activity, leading to nerve impairment and a 'cathartic' colon. There is no real evidence that healthy, active old people are much more likely to be constipated than younger people, and prophylactic laxative-taking is best avoided unless constipation is a known problem which cannot be resolved by other means. Because of some atrophy of bowel mucosa and muscle, transit times do rise somewhat with age. Elderly patients should be reassured that decreased frequency of defaecation is normal with age, and taught not to equate this with 'constipation' unless motions also become hard and difficult to pass.

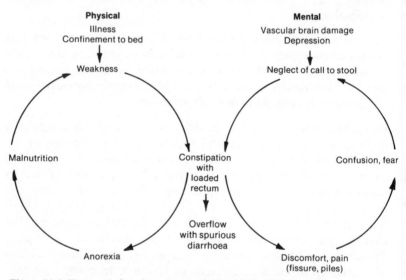

Figure 14.4 *Vicious circles of constipation in the elderly (Wilkins, 1968).*

Investigation of constipation and faecal impaction

Given the large number of possible causes outlined above, constipation with faecal impaction and incontinence should always be investigated and the underlying causes remedied, where possible. A rectal digital examination will reveal most impactions, although occasionally only soft faeces are present and the rectum may even be empty. A plain abdominal X-ray will reveal higher impaction if this is suspected. Many causes are quite easily treated, such as changing a drug regime, treating hypothyroidism or piles, or acquiring a new set of dentures so that solid food can be chewed.

Further investigation will depend on the clinical picture. Barium studies are useful if malignancy or diverticular disease are suspected.

Endoscopy of the anal canal, rectum and sigmoid colon may be useful. Blood and stool tests may be indicated. A few specialist clinics have facilities for sophisticated measurement of anal and rectal pressures, largely as a research tool at present.

Nursing assessment of the patient with suspected impaction should include a careful history of the problem (with consideration of the patient's likely reluctance to discuss it due to embarrassment, and with as much privacy as possible). Diet, mobility, fluid intake, the environment and reactions to it should all be closely observed and their relevance determined. Table 14.3 (overleaf) shows an Assessment of Defaecation checklist which the nurse might find helpful.

As well as causing incontinence, impaction can lead to intestinal obstruction, to mental disturbances (including apathy and possibly agitation or confusion), to rectal bleeding, and to urinary retention (with possible overflow incontinence).

Treatment of incontinence caused by impaction
The first necessity is to clear the faecal impaction. A manual evacuation of the faeces will rarely be necessary. More usually a course of disposable phosphate enemas, one or two per day for seven to ten days, or until no further return is obtained, is the best method of clearing impaction. A single enema is seldom sufficient, even if an apparently good result is obtained, because impaction is often very extensive and the first enema merely clears the lowest portion of the bowel. Many patients' fear of enemas stems from the days of large-volume soap-and-water enemas, which were both extremely uncomfortable and usually messy. These should no longer be used. The modern low-volume (100–150ml) disposable phosphate enema causes minimal discomfort and, if administered with careful prior explanation and due attention to privacy and dignity, does not generally cause much distress. The newer 'micro' (5–10ml) enemas are even more acceptable.

If faecal incontinence persists once the bowel has been totally cleared (a plain abdominal X-ray may be helpful to confirm this), it can usually be assumed to be neurogenic in origin rather than caused by impaction.

Once the impaction is cleared, every effort must be made to prevent recurrence. Attention to diet, fluid intake, mobility, lavatory facilities and drug regimes may be sufficient. Some patients will additionally need to use agents to keep their bowels regular. There is a huge variety of laxatives available. They can be divided into four categories:

Table 14.3: Assessment of Defaecation Checklist

Name: Assessment date:

Patient's usual term for defaecation:

Usual frequency of bowel action: Range:

Usual time of day:

Any associated habits/events:

Does patient complain of constipation?

If so, what is understood by this?

Does patient get sensation of the need to defaecate?

Average time taken for bowel action:

Does patient have to strain?

Is defaecation associated with pain?

Any bleeding?   Fresh or altered blood:

Mucus:

Problematic flatus: Continent of flatus:

Scybala: Ribbon stools:

Usual consistency of faeces:

Usual amount of faeces:

Does patient experience urgency?   Time of warning:

Diet: Any food taken for bowels?

        Any food avoided for bowels?

        Average daily fluid intake:

Laxative use: Present:

                Past history of use:

Any constipating drugs taken?

History of perianal problems:

Faecal incontinence?

If yes: Nature of soiling:

Sensation of incontinence:

Frequency of incontinence:

Result of rectal examination if done:

Any recent change in bowel habits?

Toilet facilities:

Problems with using lavatory:

If bedpan/commode used, reaction to this:

Ability to cleanse after defaecation:

Mobility impaired?

Are any bowel problems anticipated with current illness/condition?

bulking agents, stool softeners, chemical laxatives, and per rectum evacuants (Table 14.4).

Table 14.4:   Commonly-Used Laxatives

Category	Notes/Contra-indications	Examples
Bulking agents	Introduce gradually, only after impaction cleared. Avoid if patient has loss of rectal sensation or terminal reservoir syndrome	Natural bran Isogel
Stool softeners	Many (see text): avoid general use	Liquid paraffin Castor oil
Irritant/chemical	Use minimal effective dose	Senna Bisacodyl
Combined softener/ irritant	Use minimal effective dose	Dorbanex
Miscellaneous	Flatus can be problematic	Lactulose
Rectally administered	Some patients may need assistance or find use unpleasant	Suppositories (e.g. glycerine, bisacodyl) Enemas (e.g. phosphate, micro enemas)

Laxatives. The bulking laxatives work by being hydrophilic, i.e. attracting water into the stool. Usually faeces is 60–70% water, and a mere 10% increase in water content softens the stool considerably. Natural unprocessed bran is probably the most satisfactory bulking agent, but proprietary brands (e.g. Isogel) are available. Bran, because it is mixed with food and chewed, is less likely to form a bolus and therefore has a low risk of leading to intestinal obstruction. Bulking agents eaten as granules carry a slight risk of adhering together as a bolus. It must be remembered that bulking agents will take several days to reach the colon and that any impaction should be cleared before starting use. If not, the additional bulk will merely accumulate above the impaction and add to the amount of faeces which needs to be cleared. Bulking agents will increase the water content and size of stool, and decrease gut transit time, thereby increasing frequency of defaecation. They should be used with care for patients with diminished rectal sensation, those who ignore the call to stool and those with known terminal reservoir syndrome. The gradual introduction of bulking agents will tend to minimise problems.

Stool softeners are oral laxatives intended to alter stool consistency. The commonest softener was once liquid paraffin. The use of liquid paraffin should now have been discontinued as so many harmful effects have been noted, including interference with digestion, binding of fat-soluble vitamins, possible deposits in lungs from inhalation leading to lipoid pneumonia, paraffinomas (deposits in the tissues), and faecal incontinence. Likewise, castor oil should not be in general regular use as it works by stimulating the small bowel to massive activity, leading to complete bowel clearance within two hours in most people. It is therefore good for 'one-off' clearances (e.g. prior to X-ray examinations), but the water, electrolyte and nutrient loss involved make it unsuitable for repeated use, especially with the elderly.

Chemical, or irritant, laxatives work by stimulating colonic peri-stalsis. The most commonly used are senna (e.g. Senokot) and bisacodyl (as Dulcolax). As they are selective to the colon, they do not upset the whole gut and have minimal effect on fluid and electrolyte balance and gut flora. For prolonged administration, the smallest effective dose should always be used.

Dorbanex is a combination of a softener and chemical laxative and has been found to be effective in the long-term regulation of bowel function. Lactulose, a sugar, does not really fit into any category. Taken orally, it is not absorbed but attracts water and so softens the stool. Some patients find it causes a bloated feeling and excessive flatus.

Of the rectally administered laxatives the disposable small-volume enemas are probably the most convenient and effective, but their use usually necessitates help. For lesser problems glycerine or bisacodyl suppositories may be found effective and can be used independently by many people.

Often the best regime for each individual will only be found by trial and error. It is most important to prevent recurrence of impaction, or incontinence will usually return. When dealing with patients in a home or hospital this will often involve very close observation of each person's bowel habits. The traditional nursing practice of merely asking each patient if the bowels have been opened and marking 'yes' or 'no' on the TPR chart or in the Kardex is insufficient. Great vigilance is needed to avert the preventable condition of incontinence caused by impaction. The patient must be asked in more detail about the motions – their consistency, amount, ease of passage, and about any feelings of discomfort, bloating or incomplete evacuation. The nurse must respect the patient's dignity and be sensitive to likely embarrassment, and choose an opportunity of asking such questions in private. Questions asked in front of visitors or other patients are less likely to be fully answered and spontaneous comments may be discouraged. If the patient cannot be relied upon for an accurate account, it is the nurse's responsibility to observe the stool and note its characteristics herself. The difficult passage of one small hard pellet per day, which all too often is recorded as 'bowels open' and assumed to be evidence that all is well, is usually the exact opposite – a pointer to impending impaction. Where this is suspected, the nurse must perform a rectal examination to ensure that impaction is not developing. The momentary discomfort caused by a digital rectal examination is minimal compared to the distress and inconvenience resulting from faecal impaction and incontinence.

Meticulous observation, coupled with optimism and a belief that impaction is avoidable, can greatly reduce the prevalence of faecal incontinence in our caring institutions.

PREVENTION OF FAECAL INCONTINENCE

Much faecal incontinence can be prevented. Alterations to lifelong dietary habits could prevent many disorders, such as diverticular disease and possibly carcinoma, which later cause incontinence. Regular laxative use or abuse should be avoided, as it may cause colonic and nerve damage. Avoidance of straining at stool could help to preserve pelvic-floor integrity, as will better obstetric care, with a shortened second stage of labour. Public education about fluid intake, the importance of establishing a regular bowel habit, diet, and avoiding laxatives and straining could in future prevent many problems.

For those who come under the nurse's care, greater thought should go into their needs for privacy, comfort, and adequate time for defaecation. Again, the importance of diet, fluids, exercise and relevant drug regimes must be stressed. Nurses who create an environment geared to the promotion of continence, who have an attitude that this is a preventable or reversible condition, and who are prepared to make strenuous efforts to closely monitor the bowel function of all their patients, will do much to prevent the misery of faecal incontinence.

INTRACTABLE FAECAL INCONTINENCE

Protection

If faecal incontinence proves intractable for any reason, as it may be for a small minority of people, protection will be needed to preserve the sufferer's dignity and protect the environment. Many of the garments used for urinary incontinence are suitable (see Chapter 13), especially those with a disposable pad worn directly next to the perineum. If faecal incontinence alone is present, a high absorbency is usually not needed and relatively thin pads may be used. If large formed stools are passed, some people find a 'wing-folded' pad most successful at containing the stool until it can be disposed of. Marsupial pants and washable underpads (e.g. Kylie) are not suitable for faecal incontinence.

Smell

The odour of faeces is a particularly difficult problem. Obviously prompt action to dispose of the faeces and scrupulous personal hygiene (with regular baths if possible) is the best management, but even this will not always prevent smell. Proprietary deodorants such as Nilodor (Loxley), Ozium (Downs) or Atmocol (Thackray), may help if used on a pad, clothing, or in the air. Each patient may find that certain foods aggravate smell and are best avoided. Smell is one of the unsolved problems associated with faecal incontinence.

Colostomy

A person with severe persistent faecal incontinence may wish to be considered for surgical diversion of the bowel into a colostomy. The faeces can then be collected in a discreet, odour-free bag and the patient can regain social acceptability. This is, of course, very much a last resort but should not be forgotten as an alternative where incontinence is severely limiting life-style and activities. It can, with good advice and support, be a very positive decision for someone whose life is otherwise ruled by their incontinence.

FAECAL INCONTINENCE IN CHILDREN

The majority of children are continent of faeces by the age of four years, but 1% are still having problems at seven years. More boys than girls are incontinent, suggesting that developmental factors may be relevant, as boys mature more slowly.

Faecal incontinence or soiling in childhood (sometimes referred to as 'encopresis') has for long, like nocturnal enuresis, been regarded as evidence of psychiatric or psychological disorder in the child. Psychological factors are certainly very important, but it is not true that most faecally incontinent children are disturbed (Morgan, 1981).

It is not difficult to see how the incontinence arises in most cases. The child usually has fastidious, over-anxious parents who are intent upon potty-training. The child is punished for soiling, so tends to inhibit defaecation, both in the pants and in the pot. Often when attempting potty-training the child is repeatedly sat on the pot in the absence of a full rectum and simply cannot perform. The situation becomes fraught with anxiety, and bowel movements become associated with unpleasantness in the child's mind. He therefore retains faeces and becomes constipated. Defaecation is then also difficult and painful.

The tension created while on the potty or lavatory is often relieved later when out playing. 'Respite defaecation' occurs when the child relaxes – a formed stool is passed into the pants. This may seem like deliberate naughtiness to the parent who has just spent time encouraging its passage in the correct place.

Once this pattern is established, the child may even become impacted and suffer displacement incontinence or spurious diarrhoea. Tension at home or lack of privacy at school can both lead to deliberate retention. The child is made to feel guilty about his incontinence, although he has no control over it, and may try to conceal it by hiding the faeces or clothing. This may be misinterpreted as deliberate dirty habits – in fact it is rare that a child uses deliberate smearing or soiling as a weapon against parents.

The incontinent child and his parents should be assessed for their attitude to the problem. A rectal examination will reveal impaction, idiopathic megacolon or a painful fissure. Rarely, a congenital abnormality of the rectum or anus may be present. The majority of children can be treated by disimpaction of the bowel, simple explanation and reassurance, and the use by parents of simple rewards for appropriate defaecation. Punishment for soiling should not be used, as this merely aggravates the anxiety over defaecation. Neither should clean pants be rewarded, as this might reinforce retention of faeces. Regular laxatives and sensitive counselling and support will remedy most problems. Sometimes advice will include practical measures, such as the use of a footstool to support dangling legs to aid defaecation, or a lower lock that the child can reach to ensure privacy, or getting him up ten minutes earlier, so that he has time to empty the bowel before school. If, however, the child does prove to be disturbed, as a few do, then psychotherapy may be indicated.

The mentally handicapped child may be in exactly the same position as the normal child – retaining faeces because of the unfavourable response they produce in others. Conversely, incontinence may produce much commotion and attention and so become rewarding. Behaviour modification programmes of appropriate prompt rewards and gradually withdrawn prompts will cure many mentally handicapped children of incontinence (see Chapter 12). If the incontinence has a neurogenic basis (e.g. some children with spina bifida) the same constipating and planned evacuation programme as for adults may be followed.

The health visitor has an important role in educating parents to avoid many problems of faecal incontinence arising in children. Clear practical advice on potty-training, and support for those experiencing problems, will often prevent incontinence at an early stage.

FAECAL INCONTINENCE IN DEMENTIA

Severe dementia or confusional states may result in faecal incontinence caused by the loss of social awareness of what is appropriate behaviour. The person who has no conception that defaecation should only be in clearly defined receptacles has no reason to voluntarily delay defaecation, so the stool is usually passed as soon as it enters the anal canal. Sometimes the knowledge that certain receptacles are designated for the purpose is retained but the ability to identify them is lost, and the demented person may use a totally inappropriate receptacle, such as a waste-paper bin or a sink, in which to pass faeces. Others remember to remove clothing and to sit or squat, but will do so wherever they happen to be at the time. Some lose all apparent awareness and pass the stool into their underpants or the bed. Some demented people lose all appropriate toilet behaviour, but retain an appreciation that something is wrong and become agitated or start wandering, apparently aimlessly, just prior to being incontinent.

It should never be assumed that dementia alone is sufficient reason to explain faecal incontinence, without investigation and exclusion of other causes. Continence is deeply ingrained in most of us, and it is often one of the last social skills to be lost. The demented person may be incontinent because of diarrhoea from any cause; because the same neurological damage which has caused dementia has also affected the ability to voluntarily control the defaecation reflex; or, most commonly of all, because of faecal impaction. The majority of demented people are *not* faecally incontinent. Unless the dementia is profound, incontinence is most often found to have other causes.

Where the patient gives any signs of impending defaecation, there will usually be enough time to prevent incontinence by getting him to a lavatory. This is of course dependent on all those looking after that person knowing exactly what signs to look for and what they mean. Spotting this characteristic behaviour for each person is a vital part of the nursing assessment of faecal incontinence in demented people.

It may be possible to retrain the demented person to more socially acceptable habits. It is often possible to establish a routine of defaecation, for example, half an hour after a hot meal or drink. The principles of behaviour modification (see Chapters 8 and 12) are equally applicable to faecal as to urinary incontinence. Rewarding continent behaviour may restore continence in many demented people. If this is unsuccessful, the same regime as outlined for the neurogenic bowel can be used – artificial constipation alternating with planned evacuation. Naturally, such a programme requires meticulous nursing care and record-keeping to keep the patient's condition satisfactory.

REFERENCES AND FURTHER READING

Avery Jones, F., Godding, E. W., 1972. *Management of Constipation.* Blackwell Scientific Publications, Oxford and London.

Breckman, B., 1981. *Stoma Care.* Beaconsfield Publishers, Beaconsfield.

Brocklehurst, J. C., 1978. 'The Large Bowel'. In: Brocklehurst, J. C., (ed.), *Textbook of Geriatric Medicine and Gerontology* (2nd edn.). Churchill Livingstone, Edinburgh and London.

Connell, A. M., Hilton, C., Irvine, G., Lennard-Jones, J. E., Misiewicz, J. J., 1965. 'Variation of bowel habit in two population samples'. *British Medical Journal,* ii, 1095–1099.

Egan, M., Plymat, K., Thomas, T., Meade, T., 1983. 'Incontinence in patients in two district general hospitals'. *Nursing Times,* 79, 5, 22–24.

Leigh, R. J., Turnberg, L. A., 1982. 'Faecal incontinence: the unvoiced symptom'. *Lancet,* 1, 1349–1351.

Morgan, R., 1981. *Childhood Incontinence.* William Heinemann Medical Books, London.

Parks, A. G., 1980. 'Faecal Incontinence'. In: Mandelstam, D., (ed.), *Incontinence and its Management.* Croom Helm, Beckenham.

Wilkins, E. G., 1968. 'Vicious circles of constipation in the elderly'. *Postgraduate Medical Journal,* 44, 728.

Chapter 15

Catheterisation

The use of a hollow tube, or 'catheter', for urine drainage has a long history. The ancient Egyptians used gold catheters and the Greeks had bronze tubes for the relief of urinary obstruction (Cule, 1980). Modern technology has today resulted in a wide variety of catheters suitable for use in different situations. This chapter outlines how good catheter management can lead to the successful control of bladder function. Two categories of catheter are considered – the indwelling urethral (or Foley) catheter and the suprapubic catheter. (See Chapter 10 for intermittent catheter regimes.)

INDWELLING URETHRAL (FOLEY) CATHETERS

It was not until the 1930s that Frederick Foley perfected a technique for the manufacture of a one-piece catheter and balloon, by the dipping and coagulation of latex on metal forms. Today the Foley catheter is the most commonly used of all urinary catheters. In its most usual form it has a double lumen shaft (one lumen for urine drainage, the other for inflation and deflation of the balloon), a rounded tip, and two drainage eyes proximal to the balloon (Figure 15.1).

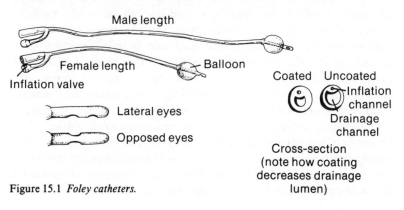

Figure 15.1 *Foley catheters.*

267

There are many variations on this standard design, both in materials and construction. Table 15.1 summarises the most common variants in use. The size of a catheter is measured on the Charrière (ch) or French gauge (f.g.) – these are in fact identical and measure the external circumference of the catheters in millimetres, usually in graduations of 2mm. A 14 f.g. catheter therefore has an external circumference of 14mm.

INDICATIONS FOR AN INDWELLING URETHRAL CATHETER

There are many situations in which an indwelling urethral catheter may be used. In the acute hospital setting, post-operative drainage, particularly after urological or gynaecological surgery, and during severe illness where accurate monitoring of urine output is needed, are the commonest indications. Chronic or acute retention of urine is often managed by catheter, either short-term until the retention is treated, or long-term if treatment is impossible or unsuccessful. The terminally ill may benefit from the use of a catheter if bladder management becomes a problem, either because of incontinence (which is distressing, difficult to manage, and can cause severe skin problems), or because micturition has become too frequent, too painful, or too difficult for the patient's comfort. A catheter may make the difference between relatives being able to cope at home, and the dying person needing hospital care.

Intractable urinary incontinence, from any cause, may also be managed by an indwelling catheter. This, it must be stressed, should be very much a last resort, and a catheter should never be the first line of management for incontinence. But if, after full investigation and a trial of available treatments, the person remains so incontinent that the quality of his life is impaired and a normal life-style is impossible in reasonable comfort and dignity, a catheter can be a very positive method of management. Patients who are too unwell or frail to undergo therapy for incontinence may also benefit. Insertion of a catheter to control incontinence should only proceed after full discussion of the implications between doctor, patient, nurse and relevant others (e.g. relatives), when all agree and accept the decision. A catheter should never be inserted for the convenience of staff; it must always be a decision taken for the well-being of the patient. For the severely incontinent, a catheter may be the only way of being socially acceptable, and for some it may allow an independent life free from the need for institutionalised care, or allow care by relatives who otherwise could not or would not cope with incontinence at home. For

Table 15.1: Types of Foley Catheter

STANDARD MALE-LENGTH FOLEY CATHETER
Length: 40–45 cm
Balloon sizes: 3ml (child), 5ml, 5–10ml, 30ml
Sizes: 8–30 f.g. in 2mm graduations
Material
- Plastic – short-term
- Latex rubber – short-term
- Siliconised – provides lubrication for insertion
- Teflon-coated – long-term
- Silicone elastomer-coated latex – long-term
- 100% silicone – long-term

FEMALE-LENGTH FOLEY CATHETER
Length: 20–25 cm
Balloon sizes: 5ml, 5–10ml, 30ml
Sizes: 12–26 f.g.
Material
- Latex rubber – short-term
- Teflon-coated – long-term
- Silicone elastomer-coated latex – long-term
- 100% silicone – long-term

ROBERTS CATHETER
Length: 40 cm
Balloon sizes: 5ml
Sizes: 12–24 f.g.
Material
- Teflon-coated – one eye below balloon for drainage

DOUBLE BALLOON
Length: 40 cm
Balloon sizes: 5–10ml, 30ml
Sizes: 16 f.g.
Material
- Latex rubber – double balloon for women – one each at internal and external meatus to prevent movement

3-WAY CATHETER
Length: 40–45 cm
Balloon sizes: 5–10ml, 30–50ml, 75–100 ml
Sizes: 18–26 f.g.
Material
- Plastic or latex-rubber – some reinforced to prevent collapse with suction. For continuous irrigation

women who have no alternative to the absorbent pad, and for men who cannot use an appliance, a well-managed catheter can restore social continence and a full range of normal activities.

SELECTION OF THE CATHETER

Once the decision to use an indwelling catheter has been made, the choice of catheter type is crucial. With the comfort and well-being of the patient at stake it is not acceptable merely to use the first catheter that comes to hand from the store cupboard. Whoever is inserting the catheter should be aware of the range available and their different intended functions.

Size

The golden rule when selecting catheter size is to choose the smallest catheter that will drain adequately. For an adult this will normally be a 12, 14, or 16 f.g. Size 8 f.g. catheters are the smallest available for children, and for infants an infant feeding tube may be used. Except where heavy haematuria is anticipated, sizes larger than 18 f.g. should never be used for initial catheterisation in adults, and indeed larger sizes are almost never indicated, even after prolonged catheterisation, unless excessive amounts of debris are present. It is all too common for patients presenting with a problematic catheter to have a large catheter in situ (up to 28 f.g.), which has been inserted by an inexperienced person. The purpose of a catheter is *not* to occlude the urethra completely, like a cork in a bottle neck. The folds of the urethra normally close upon themselves, and the smaller the catheter the more easily the urethral folds can close around it.

Except at the sphincters there should be adequate space around the catheter so that secretions from the paraurethral glands can drain. If these glands are occluded the secretions accumulate and tend to become infected, which can lead to an abscess or to stricture formation (Figure 15.2).

A catheter which is too large will also risk causing a urethral pressure sore in men, either where it is gripped at the external sphincter or where it bends over the penoscrotal junction (Blandy, 1981). This may be followed by sloughing granuloma and stricture formation (Figure 15.3). This is not uncommonly seen after major non-urological surgery (e.g. cardiac surgery), where an inexperienced person has inserted a very large catheter for the purposes of post-operative urinary output monitoring. The patient may recover well from his original complaint but be left with a problematic urethral stricture.

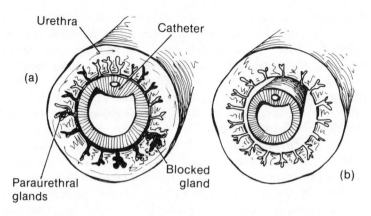

Figure 15.2 *The importance of catheter size.* (a) *Too large a catheter blocks drainage from the paraurethral glands.* (b) *A smaller catheter permits secretions to drain (Blandy, 1981).*

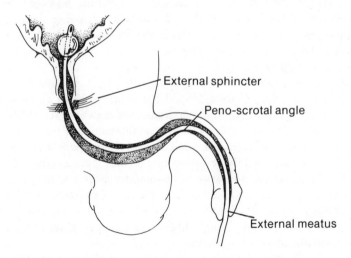

Figure 15.3 *Sites for catheter stricture (Blandy, 1981).*

Larger catheters do not necessarily have larger eyes in proportion, so will often block just as easily as smaller ones. Coated catheters have an especially small eye and lumen size in proportion to their f.g. size (Figure 15.1).

271

Balloon size

Manufacturers indicate on their packaging of a catheter the maximum amount of fluid with which a balloon should be filled – usually 5ml, 5–10ml or 30ml. Very large balloons (75ml and over) are intended specifically for controlling post-operative haematuria and should not be used for general purposes. The stated amount is commonly misinterpreted as the amount that *must* be used in that balloon rather than as a maximum capacity. A custom has grown up in the UK of using 30ml balloon catheters, filled with 30ml of water, as standard practice for routine drainage. This large amount is certainly unnecessary, except in certain cases – for instance, where the bladder neck has been damaged – and is the cause of many catheter-associated problems. In the USA the 5ml balloon is used routinely, and this practice is currently gaining acceptance in the UK. A larger balloon is seldom necessary to hold a catheter in place. If the only catheter available has a stated balloon capacity of 30ml, it is possible to use much less water (e.g. 15ml) to retain it – although less than this will lead to uneven balloon inflation. The balloon is not designed to occlude the internal urethral meatus to prevent leakage (this is prevented by the bladder neck and sphincters gripping the catheter lumen), but merely to gently retain the catheter in the bladder to prevent it from falling out. Few patients need more than 5–10ml of fluid for this purpose.

One major problem caused by using too large a balloon is the bypassing or leakage of urine around the catheter. With all catheters, except the Roberts catheter, the drainage eyes are above the balloon. If a 5ml balloon is used this results in a small amount of residual urine, which is unable to escape, being left around the balloon. If the balloon has 30ml of water in it the residual urine volume is much larger (Figure 15.4). The larger balloon irritates the bladder more and may provoke contractions, especially in an unstable bladder. Contractions will force the residual urine out around the catheter, and the larger the residue, the greater the potential for leakage. The larger residual also has an increased likelihood of infection.

Thirty millilitres of water is also heavy, especially when resting on the delicate and sensitive trigone of the bladder. This can lead to feelings of discomfort or dragging with a catheter. Also, if for some reason there is repeated traction or pulling on the catheter, this weight may damage the bladder neck. It is sometimes stated that a large balloon is necessary to prevent confused patients from pulling the catheter out. However, it is certainly not unknown for a patient to pull

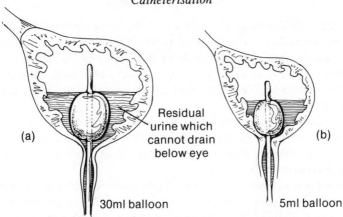

Figure 15.4 *Balloon catheters.* (a) *30ml balloon.* (b) *5–10ml balloon.*

out a fully inflated 30ml balloon, and if there is a likelihood of the patient pulling the catheter out, it is infinitely preferable to pull out a smaller rather than a larger balloon – the additional discomfort from pulling out a larger balloon is seldom a deterrent to the confused patient. Indeed the weight and discomfort caused by a 30ml balloon in the bladder may be the cause of the pulling. Repeated traction upon a smaller balloon is less likely to damage the bladder neck. Some nursing texts recommend restraining or using mittens on the confused catheterised patient. The ethics of this seem dubious and it is better to avoid the use of a catheter if a confused or uncooperative patient tends to pull at it.

Catheter material

Until relatively recently, most catheters were made either from plastic (polyvinylchloride or polyurethane) or latex rubber. Red rubber has on occasion been used, but it tends to be very irritant and the incidence of adverse reaction is high. Plastic is soft at body temperature but rigid at lower temperatures and is often found by women to be uncom-fortable, especially when sitting. Both plastic and latex rubber tend to develop cracks and encrustations with prolonged use (after about two weeks). Plastic possibly attracts less encrustation because its negative surface electrical charge discourages particle adhesion, although the clinical results of this are unproven. Both plastic and latex catheters are relatively cheap.

Many attempts have been made to improve upon the latex catheter to prolong its life, reduce encrustation and infection, and improve comfort. 'Siliconising' the surface of the latex catheter produces a lubricated surface, which is said to ease insertion and provide some lubrication while the catheter is in situ. The coating dissolves after insertion which, as lubricant jelly is always also used, is seldom a problem anyway. The extra cost of siliconised catheters is thus of debatable value.

Latex can be coated with teflon, which is claimed to make the latex inert and to give a smoother surface. This may reduce urethritis and stone formation, although there is no clear evidence that teflon reduces encrustation.

Many extravagant claims have been made for catheters coated or dipped in silicone elastomer ('silicone-coated', which should be distinguished from the 'siliconised' catheters described above). There does seem to be less encrustation with silicone-coated than latex catheters in long-term use, and some reduction in tissue reaction. Some manufacturers claim that they can safely be left in situ for three to six months without changing. Latex has been found to be equally long-lasting if well managed (Blannin and Hobden, 1980). It is possible that encrustation itself is not a major factor in catheter life-span, and many are changed for other reasons – especially leakage – long before encrustation has become a problem. If silicone-coated catheters are not used for their full intended life-span, it must be questioned whether they are worth their considerable extra cost (often five to six times that of a latex catheter). It has yet to be determined whether the reduced lumen from the coating actually impairs drainage, encourages blockage, and shortens the catheter's life.

More recently, 100% silicone catheters have been introduced. As they are not coated, the internal lumen tends to be proportionately larger. However, because silicone permits gas diffusion they tend to have problems with balloon deflation over time. Without close supervision some patients find the catheter falls out before its expected life is over.

On current evidence it seems best to choose a cheap catheter (plastic or latex) for first or short-term use. If this is well tolerated, without problems for an initial two-week trial period, the additional cost of a silicone-coated or all-silicone catheter is justified. If well managed, this will remain in place for at least three months. If the patient experiences repeated problems which necessitate frequent catheter changes, then a latex or plastic catheter is more cost-effective, as the more expensive catheters have no proven advantages in short-term use. Indeed, some people find latex suitable for long-term use.

Catheter design

For most purposes, a man will be catheterised with a standard male-length catheter and a woman with a female-length catheter with a 5ml or 5–10ml balloon. Many nurses are unaware of the existence of female-length catheters. There is no reason to use the longer catheters for most women – their greater length makes them difficult to disguise under clothing and easier to pull accidentally. If thigh drainage is used, they are also more likely to form a loop, which means that urine has to drain uphill into the drainage bag.

The Roberts catheter, which has one eye below the balloon, may be of use when leakage is a problem, e.g. with the unstable bladder. Urine which normally would not be able to drain may be squeezed out of the distal eye, rather than around the catheter by bladder contractions.

Most catheters have a semi-rigid rounded tip. Variations include the Tiemann tip, which is curved to aid insertion past an enlarged prostate, and whistle tip which is open-ended to facilitate drainage of debris. Most catheters have two drainage eyes. These may be lateral (on the same side) or opposed (on opposite sides, which is possibly less likely to block, Figure 15.1).

INSERTION OF AN INDWELLING CATHETER

The decision to institute drainage by indwelling catheter is a medical one and should always be made by the responsible medical practitioner. The actual insertion should be done by a nurse or doctor who has received full instruction and who has had supervised practice in the technique. There is little obvious reason for the tradition that doctors or male nurses catheterise men, and female nurses catheterise women. So long as local chaperoning regulations are followed, any competent professional should be able to catheterise any patient.

When the insertion of an indwelling catheter is not done in the operating theatre, it should always be done using strict aseptic technique, whether in the home or in hospital (Bielski, 1980). In most situations pre-packed catheter packs are available. The importance of selecting the right catheter has already been stressed. Ideally, the patient should have a bath prior to catheter insertion. If this is not possible, a thorough wash of the genital area with soap and water is essential.

For women, the key to successful catheter insertion lies in visualising the urethral meatus clearly. The patient should lie semi-recumbent with knees bent and abducted to either side as far as possible. An angle-poise light directed at the vulva can be very helpful. A cotton bud will help to locate the meatus if it is disguised among skin folds. If the opening is concealed it may be easier to find with the patient in the left lateral position with her knees drawn up onto her chest, so that the anterior vaginal wall can be visualised from behind.

In men the foreskin should be retracted and the glans penis thoroughly cleaned. Local anaesthetic gel (e.g. Lignocaine 1%) must be instilled into the penis using an applicator and then held in by gentle pressure, using either the fingers or a penile clamp, for at least four minutes. The catheter is inserted extending the penis vertically with gentle but firm lateral grasp. If resistance is met at the external sphincter, the patient is asked to relax and pretend to pass urine. The usual reason for encountering resistance at this point is insufficient anaesthesia. The catheter should never be forced in, but withdrawn and some more anaesthetic instilled before re-inserting the catheter after a further four minutes. Catheter-introducers are dangerous in inexperienced hands and should only be used by a trained urologist. When the catheter still fails to pass, a smaller or softer one may be tried. If this fails, urological assistance should be sought. When the catheter is in situ the foreskin must be replaced.

Most health authorities have their own detailed procedures laid down for catheterisation, and these should be consulted and followed.

DRAINAGE BAGS

Once a catheter has been inserted it should immediately be connected to a drainage bag. The type of bag will be selected according to the needs of the individual patient. Most bags have a non-return valve at their inlet to prevent urine refluxing once it has entered the bag. Bags without this valve should not be used with an indwelling catheter.

The patient who is bed-bound or receiving continuous bladder irrigation will usually need a 2-litre capacity bag, which can be supported by a bed-hanger or floor-stand. These bags are also used for a short-term catheter and for overnight drainage with a long-term catheter.

Ambulant patients, especially those whose catheter is to be in for more than a few days, will need a smaller body-worn bag for use by day. It is not acceptable to oblige a patient to carry around a 2-litre bag of urine like a handbag, in full view. The most usual body-worn bag is the leg bag. This may have a capacity of 350ml, 500ml, or 750ml, and is secured to the leg with straps which may be made from latex, fabric ties, elastic or foam rubber and Velcro. Leg-straps can cause problems if too tight (a full bag can be heavy), and some people develop a sensitivity to latex. The inlet may be short, for thigh-wearing, or longer to wear over the knee or on the calf (under trousers). The calf-bag is emptied by lifting up the bottom of the trousers. A thigh-bag can be emptied more easily if a small Velcro-fastened opening is made in the inner trouser seam.

Alternatively, a drainage bag may be suspended from a waist-belt, 'sporran' style (Figure 15.5). These bags hold up to 1 litre and have side inlets to prevent kinking. As the weight is more evenly distributed, many patients find this more comfortable than leg-straps. Very obese patients may find that the waist-belt does not stay up easily, and the immobile must take care that the bag is below bladder level. Women find the sporran particularly useful under skirts, since there is no danger, as there is with a leg bag, of the bag sliding down and becoming visible.

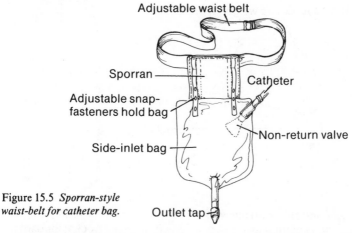

Figure 15.5 *Sporran-style waist-belt for catheter bag.*

Drainage bags, whether small or large, can be held in specially designed garments (pants, trousers, or skirts) with an integral pocket for the bag (Fig. 15.6, overleaf). The plastic of the bag is not in contact with the skin, and even a 2-litre bag can be kept discreetly out of sight.

The selection of an outlet tap, which the patient can manage easily, is important. Some bags have a removable rubber cap which is easily dropped, possibly down the lavatory, and is obviously unsuitable for those with poor manual dexterity. Some people find a push-pull valve easy, others prefer a twist-and-pull type. Larger taps are often easier to manage, but may dig into the leg. Some taps are now available which

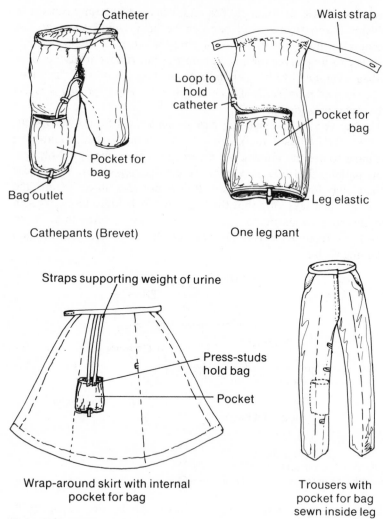

Catheter

Waist strap

Loop to hold catheter

Pocket for bag

Pocket for bag

Bag outlet

Leg elastic

Cathepants (Brevet)

One leg pant

Straps supporting weight of urine

Press-studs hold bag

Pocket

Wrap-around skirt with internal pocket for bag

Trousers with pocket for bag sewn inside leg

Figure 15.6 *Leg bag garments.*

allow a night-drainage bag to be connected directly to the bottom of the smaller day bag without breaking the system (Figure 15.7). These can be used with cheap sterile non-drainable (single-use) bags in hospital, or with ordinary drainable bags which can be washed out at home.

Some bags now incorporate a quilting to spread the urine more evenly and allow the bag to conform to the contour of the leg.

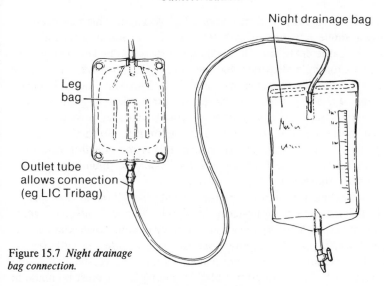

Night drainage bag

Leg bag

Outlet tube allows connection (eg LIC Tribag)

Figure 15.7 *Night drainage bag connection.*

INFECTION AND THE INDWELLING CATHETER

The normal urinary tract has several defences against infection. Complete bladder emptying, the regular scouring action of micturition, and a competent sphincter mechanism all help to prevent bacterial invasion and to eradicate any micro-organisms promptly and completely. The introduction of an indwelling catheter into this normally sterile system provides three potential entry portals for infection: on the catheter itself during insertion, around the outside of the catheter via the urethra, and ascent up the lumen of the catheter. The first portal can be largely discounted if strict aseptic technique is used for insertion. The second is more of a problem in the short female urethra, but defences can be bolstered by ensuring that the catheter is small enough to allow free drainage of urethral secretions.

Ascending infection, via the catheter lumen, was the major source of infection in catheterised patients until the early 1960s. Prior to that, catheters were maintained on 'open drainage' with the end of the catheter open and draining into a non-sterile vessel. With this system, almost all catheterised bladders were infected within three to four days of insertion. Although this could be reduced, to some extent, by continuous antiseptic irrigation, infection rates remained high until the introduction of closed urinary drainage directly from the catheter into sterile sealed bags. This introduction of closed drainage has moved the point at which nearly all (98%) of catheterised bladders are infected, from four to thirty days after insertion. This has been the biggest single advance in catheter care. It has meant that infection rates for catheters in situ for less than five days can be kept below 10% in most situations, provided that the closed system is never interrupted (i.e. the catheter is never disconnected from the bag). However, beyond the 5-day point an increasing proportion of patients with catheters acquire a urinary tract infection, whatever precautions are taken, until nearly all are infected at one month. No method has yet been found which significantly reduces this rising infection rate from five to thirty days, except keeping the system scrupulously uninterrupted in the short term. Irrigation, routine washouts, systematic antibiotics and antimicrobals in the drainage bag all fail to alter this.

Catheters in situ long-term inevitably become infected. Most commonly the micro-organisms are from the patients' own commensals (e.g. *E.Coli*), but almost any organism can invade the catheterised bladder, including more exotic bacteria, fungi and yeasts. A decision to use a catheter for long-term bladder management must be made in the knowledge of the inevitability of infection.

Does this infection associated with catheters matter? One in ten patients admitted to an acute hospital will have an indwelling catheter at some point during their admission. Forty per cent of all nosocomial (hospital-acquired) infections are urinary tract infections, and 70% of these are associated with the use of an indwelling catheter. There is some evidence that those patients catheterised during admission are likely to have a longer stay in hospital, suffer more complications, and possibly have a higher incidence of fatal outcome to their hospital stay, than patients with similar illness but no catheter (Platt et al., 1982). The incidence of Gram-negative bacteraemias following catheterisation is low, but when it occurs it causes a 40% mortality. Those patients who are catheterised because they are acutely ill or have had urinary tract surgery are especially vulnerable to risks of serious complications.

If the catheter is likely to be in place short-term, it is certainly worth every effort to prevent or treat infection. Once the catheter is a permanent feature, infection has to be accepted. Most of the evidence about the effects of infection from long-term catheters comes from patients with spinal injury. Many of these patients do suffer renal impairment; indeed, renal failure is the most common reason for death, apart from injury-related causes, and many are found to have scarred kidneys with pus on post-mortem examination (Warren et al., 1981).

MANAGEMENT OF THE SHORT-TERM INDWELLING CATHETER

For the short-term catheter (intended duration up to one month) the primary aim of management is to prevent urinary tract infection. The first question must always be, 'Is this catheter really necessary?' Surprisingly often the answer is 'No'. If the catheter is suggested because the patient has failed to pass urine (e.g. post-operatively), it may be possible to promote spontaneous voiding by ensuring that the patient is not in pain and has adequate privacy and comfort to pass urine, preferably on a lavatory or commode. Running taps, plenty of time and a hot cup of tea work well for many patients. How many catheters have been passed because the patient was too uncomfortable or inhibited to perform perched on a bedpan? If voiding is not achieved in the presence of a distended bladder or discomfort, an in-out catheter should usually be used in the first instance. Only after spontaneous voiding has failed to occur after several in-out catheters should an indwelling catheter be considered.

In male patients who must have their urinary output closely monitored, but who are incontinent, a penile sheath is preferable to a catheter, provided that the bladder is emptying completely.

After much urological or gynaecological surgery, a suprapubic catheter is preferable to a urethral one because the catheter can be clamped while the patient tries to void, and simply unclamped if he fails (see pages 292–294). This overcomes the problem of repeated catheter withdrawal and re-insertion in situations when some voiding problem is common. Some hospitals still use catheters routinely in certain situations (e.g. orthopaedic surgery) without consideration of individual needs and the risks involved.

If a urethral catheter is really necessary for short-term use, the duration of catheterisation must always be kept to an absolute minimum – preferably less than five days. A closed system between the catheter and bag must be maintained if at all possible. If a break is essential (e.g. to wash out a blocked catheter), then strict aseptic technique must be observed. If the need for irrigation is anticipated (e.g. post-prostatectomy), it is best to insert a three-way irrigating catheter, remembering that the junction between irrigating fluid and catheter is another break in the system and must also be treated aseptically.

The drainage bag should be emptied at least once every eight hours, using a 'no-touch' technique and a clean jug for each patient. Handwashing before *and* after any handling of the catheter or bag is very important and helps to prevent cross-infection. For the same reason, the bag should always be on a hanger and never allowed to touch the floor. Physically separating catheterised patients in a ward and, when possible, isolating those who develop an infection (e.g. in a single room), can also help to prevent cross-infection.

Catheter care, for both short-term and long-term catheters, should involve careful washing of the genital area with soap and water at least twice per day. When possible, a bath should be taken (using only soap and avoiding additives). In men, the foreskin should be retracted, the glans penis cleaned and the foreskin replaced. The genital area should then be dried thoroughly on a clean soft towel. Talcum powder should be avoided as it can clog around the catheter and irritate. Careful washing should also be encouraged after each bowel movement, and women must be instructed on correct perineal cleaning (i.e. using toilet paper from front to back, away from the catheter). Using antiseptic solutions for catheter care has no proven value and in some cases (e.g. povidone iodine) has been found to increase infection rates. Where the patient has any discharge of blood or mucus around the catheter, this should be carefully cleaned away using sterile cotton wool and water if necessary.

Bladder washouts should not be used as a routine in short-term catheter management. They have no role in preventing infection and they provide a break in the system to allow an opportunity for bacterial invasion. Likewise, systemic antibiotics have no place in the prevention of infection, and may indeed provoke the emergence of antibiotic-resistant strains, but they should be used appropriately to treat infection in short-term catheters.

Drainage bags should not be changed routinely on short-term catheters. If the bag becomes clogged with debris, a new one can be substituted using aseptic technique; otherwise most bags will last up to two weeks.

Urine specimens from catheters

The closed system does not need to be broken in taking a urine specimen from the catheter for microbiological examination, as most bags have a self-sealing sample port on the drainage tubing. The tubing should be clamped just below the port, and left for several minutes for urine to accumulate above the clamp. The sample port should be cleaned with 70% alcohol (e.g. an injection swab). The specimen is taken using a sterile needle and syringe, inserted via the sample port at an angle (to avoid going straight through the tubing and possibly injecting the nurse's fingers with infected urine). The urine should never be squirted into a specimen pot via the needle, since this can destroy any cells or casts present. The needle should always be removed first. Specimens should be taken routinely every two to three days from patients with a short-term catheter.

If a patient is gravely ill with a catheter in place, and a septicaemia originating from the bladder is suspected, a urine specimen should be obtained directly from the bladder by suprapubic aspiration, as a specimen obtained via the catheter will disagree, in one-third of all cases, with a specimen from the bladder itself. Septicaemia is a life-threatening situation which merits immediate attention.

Urine specimens should *never* be taken from the drainage bag. Wherever possible the specimen should be delivered to the laboratory within one hour of sampling, or else kept at 4°C until it can be delivered.

LONG-TERM INDWELLING CATHETER MANAGEMENT

As stated above, the use of a long-term catheter can be a very positive decision in patient management, but it must always be made bearing the risks of infection in mind. The likely benefits and costs should be considered for each patient individually. For younger patients with prolonged management by catheter, renal problems become a major cause of morbidity and mortality (Warren et al., 1981). This matters less when a patient is elderly or has a limited life expectancy. For younger patients, who may need a catheter for decades, every possible alternative should be seriously considered (e.g. suprapubic catheters, intermittent catheterisation, or urinary diversion via an ileal conduit).

The long-term catheter in a hospitalised patient should be managed in much the same way as the short-term catheter, but in the knowledge that infection probably cannot be prevented and will only be treated if the patient becomes unwell. Hospitals are prone to harbour multi-resistant organisms, and the aim must be to minimise cross-infection and to take the microbiologist's advice on sensible antimicrobal prescribing.

Home management of the long-term catheter is inevitably different. It is often impossible for rigorous asepsis to be adhered to, and it is indeed largely unnecessary in the home as organisms are likely to be the patient's own commensals. The most important factor in successful home management is that the patient, or his relatives, should fully understand how to look after the catheter. A fearful patient, afraid to touch the catheter, will be far less successful than the confident patient. To this end ample time must always be given for the newly catheterised patient to discuss any worries, and careful instruction is vital. An information sheet is useful for later reference (see Table 15.2 for an example).

The patient must be shown and given supervised practice in caring for his catheter. This includes instruction on twice-daily washing, changing day and night bags, how to empty the bag, and how to wash bags out. It is not necessary to use sterile drainage bags in the home, provided that good handwashing is employed. The bag is changed to a body-worn bag for daytime and a larger bedside bag at night. After each change, the bag is washed in warm soapy water (e.g. using washing-up liquid) and then hung up to dry. Each bag can be used for at least one week, often longer if there is little debris.

The patient is asked to drink plenty of fluid (at least two litres per day), to take reasonable exercise to avoid debris accumulation, and to avoid constipation.

Table 15.2: Home Management of a Catheter

INSTRUCTIONS TO PATIENT

The catheter is a hollow tube which will drain your urine from the bladder into a bag. You will not need to pass water yourself. These simple instructions will help you to look after your catheter properly.

1) Wash the area around your bladder outlet and the catheter thoroughly twice a day. This should be done with plain (unscented) soap and warm water and the area dried thoroughly on a soft towel. When possible a daily bath is recommended. Avoid use of talcum powder in the area. Also wash area thoroughly after a bowel motion.

2) Drink at least 4 pints (2 litres) of fluid in every 24 hours. This means about 1 cupful of liquid per hour when you are awake.

3) Wear the smaller bag when you are up and the larger bag at night. Always wash your hands thoroughly *before* and *after* changing the bags.

4) Each bag will last about 1 week. After changing each bag wash it thoroughly in warm water with a mild detergent solution (e.g. washing-up liquid). A small funnel is useful to help fill the bag with fluid. Then hang it up to dry before next use. After 1 week throw the bag away and use a new one.

5) When possible take regular daily exercise.

6) Avoid constipation as this can prevent the catheter draining properly. If constipation is a problem ask your nurse for advice.

7) Avoid bending or kinking the catheter tubing. Always keep the bag below bladder level to ensure good drainage.

Some Common Problems

1) Bladder spasms or cramps in the abdomen are common when a new catheter has been inserted. They are nothing to worry about and usually pass off within one day. If they persist, tell your nurse.

2) If no urine drains for several hours:
   – is the tubing bent or kinked?
   – is the bag below the bladder level?
   – is the bag connected the right way up?
   – have you been drinking enough?
   – are you constipated?
   – try moving or walking around as this may dislodge a blockage.

   If 4 hours or longer pass and no urine has drained, call your nurse.

3) If your catheter leaks this is not serious but should be reported to your nurse in office hours (9 a.m.–5 p.m.).

4) If the catheter falls out call your nurse in office hours if you can pass urine. If you cannot pass urine yourself and the bladder becomes painful, seek immediate help.

5) If you see blood in the urine do not worry but report it at the nurse's next visit. If the bleeding is heavy report it during office hours.

6) If your catheter is causing you problems during sexual intercourse, do not hesitate to discuss this with your nurse.

> Your nurse is:
> Address:
> Telephone No.   Office hours (9 a.m.–5 p.m.):
> Emergency No. for other times:

Please feel free to discuss any problems or queries you may have about your catheter with your nurse.

CATHETER-ASSOCIATED PROBLEMS

Catheter cramps

Most people experience abdominal cramps (often likened by women to menstrual pains) when a catheter is first inserted. A mild analgesic and simple reassurance that this is nothing to worry about will settle this within twenty-four hours for most patients. If cramps persist and are troublesome, the cause is usually an unstable bladder with contractions being experienced as discomfort. Sometimes a smaller catheter or a smaller balloon will stop this. Propantheline (15mg t.d.s.) is usually the most effective remedy. In some people the cramps are so severe as to make catheterisation inappropriate, and another form of management has to be used.

Urethral discomfort

Some urethral discomfort is common with an indwelling catheter, and this often has to be accepted. Silicone or silicone-coated catheters are said by some to be more comfortable than plastic or latex. The discomfort may be caused by too large a catheter mechanically distending the urethra, or occluding the paraurethral glands, leading to infection, urethritis, and an offensive discharge around the catheter. A smaller catheter should resolve this.

In postmenopausal women discomfort may be caused by atrophic urethritis, and a course of oestrogen replacement therapy will relieve the discomfort (see Chapter 8).

Leaking catheters

One of the most common reasons for catheter failure and premature change is leakage or by-passing. It is present in up to 40% of all patients with a catheter and is the reason for one-third of unplanned catheter changes (Kennedy and Brocklehurst, 1982; Kennedy et al., 1983). This is particularly irksome if the catheter was instituted to control incontinence, as the patient is not only still wet but also has the additional problem of catheter care.

A leaking catheter is usually caused by an unstable bladder. The bladder is irritated by the presence of the catheter and contracts uninhibitedly, squeezing urine out around the lumen of the catheter. Often using a smaller catheter or less water in the balloon decreases the irritation and thus the leakage. Also, with a smaller balloon there is less residual urine available to leak (see pages 272–273). If a catheter leaks, firstly some fluid should be taken out of the balloon, and if that does not help, a smaller catheter may be tried. Anticholinergic medication may also help to dampen the contractions (propantheline is again useful here).

The catheter may be leaking because it is blocked. Flushing the catheter out with 50ml of sterile water may unblock the catheter (in hospital this can be done aseptically via the sample port by clamping the tubing below the port). Alternatively, it may be blocked because of kinked tubing or because the bag has been consistently above bladder level.

Some patients find a Roberts catheter helps to prevent leakage (see page 275).

Haematuria
Small amounts of blood in the urine of catheterised patients is common and of no importance. It is usually caused by trauma and infection. If haematuria becomes heavy and persistent, urological advice should be sought.

Infection
In the patient with a long-term catheter, infection is both inevitable and, in most cases, asymptomatic. It is futile to treat these infections as the urine is usually only cleared for a few days, if at all (Brocklehurst and Brocklehurst, 1978), and there is a danger of more pathogenic organisms invading the bladder, or of resistance developing. Prophylactic antibiotics or antimicrobal washouts have no place in catheter management.

However, if the patient becomes ill the infection will have to be treated. Symptoms may include fever, rigors, loin pain, significant haematuria, and, in the elderly, the unexplained sudden onset of confusion. The catheter may have to be removed for treatment to be successful.

Erosion of the bladder wall
If a catheter is on continuous drainage, the tip of the catheter is always in contact with the bladder wall and may cause ulcers in the mucosa. There is some evidence that prolonged use of a catheter predisposes to bladder malignancies, and chronic irritation may be implicated. Intermittent catheter release may be used to overcome this irritation. The catheter is clamped or spigoted and released at specified intervals (Ferrie et al., 1979). Both LIC and Squibb market specially designed spigots for this use. It is usual to employ 3- to 4-hourly release by day and leave the catheter on continuous drainage overnight. This is said to reduce erosion, maintain bladder capacity, and lessen catheter

blockage by giving it a good flush out periodically. It also dispenses with the need to wear a bag, as the catheter can be emptied directly into a lavatory. This management is obviously not suitable for those with low-capacity unstable bladders, as leakage would occur between catheter releases. It is, however, a viable method for those who need a catheter because of voiding difficulties, and it deserves increased evaluation in future.

Encrustation, stones and debris

Infection and secretions mean that most patients with a long-term catheter have some debris in their urine. This is a particular problem in the immobile, as debris accumulates and can eventually block the drainage eyes. Hence patients are encouraged to be as mobile as possible. If the patient cannot move, regular passive changes of position are recommended.

All indwelling catheters become encrusted to some extent. The use of silicone or silicone-coated catheters may lessen this, but does not prevent encrustation. It can affect the lumen and eyes of the catheter by blocking them, and may make the balloon difficult to deflate. Some bacteria, notably proteus, produce the urea-splitting enzyme urease. When urease splits urea, it releases ammonia and free hydrogen ions. This process encourages the precipitation of salts from urine, classically the three phosphates of ammonium, calcium and magnesium. Stones may form around the nucleus of clumps of bacteria, or encrustation accumulate around the catheter. Once stones are present it is impossible to eradicate infection and the stones may cause pain or bleeding, or block the catheter. In immobile patients, re-uptake of calcium from the bones may make more calcium available in the urine for stone formation.

Some patients seem more prone to debris, stones or encrustation than others. A few are inveterate catheter-blockers and for these people it is worth increasing fluid intake up to three litres per day, if tolerated. For habitual blockers, regular prophylactic washouts can prevent blockage (Brocklehurst and Brocklehurst, 1978). This is best done with 50–100ml sterile water (tap water in the home) three times weekly (more often if necessary). Often a sensible patient or a relative can be taught to do this themselves.

If a patient repeatedly blocks a catheter there is no point in using expensive catheters, and a latex catheter on regular routine changes may have to be used (e.g. every two weeks). Alternatively, another form of management may have to be considered.

No drainage

If a catheter has failed to drain any urine, or only minimal amounts, over a period of several hours, the cause should be investigated. Normally urine arrives in the bladder continuously, so it should drain continuously. Sometimes the explanation is that the drainage tube has been inadvertently left clamped, or is kinked. The bag may be overfull and will not admit further urine. A rectal examination may reveal that faecal impaction is interfering with catheter drainage.

The catheter may be blocked. It can be gently rolled between two fingers and encrustations may be felt. A bladder washout may unblock the lumen or eyes. Fifty millilitres of sterile water can be instilled and allowed to drain back. If nothing returns, further increments of 50ml can be added, up to a maximum of 200ml (unless of course the patient is already experiencing discomfort or an overdistended bladder). The water should not be removed by the suction of a syringe, because the walls of the catheter can collapse and occlude the lumen completely and the bladder mucosa may be sucked into the drainage eye. If a washout fails to unblock the catheter it should be removed and replaced. The removed catheter should be inspected for the site and type of blockage. If the second catheter fails to drain, the patient may be genuinely anuric. Provided that he is not dehydrated this is a sign of renal failure, and urgent medical attention must be obtained.

Sexual activity

Sexual intercourse is possible for both men and women with a urethral catheter in situ. Men are usually advised to tape the catheter back along the shaft of the penis. However, it is not a practice to be generally recommended as discomfort is usual for both partners, and haemorrhage may occur. Considerable trauma to the urethra is inevitable, and repeated intercourse with a catheter in situ may cause eventual stricture formation. Intercourse will also not be the pleasurable activity it should be. Urethral catheters are probably best avoided for the sexually active person (never forgetting that this includes the elderly as well as the young), and alternatives such as a suprapubic catheter should be considered, especially for men. If a urethral catheter is necessary it may be feasible to teach the patient or his partner to remove the catheter prior to intercourse and insert a new one afterwards. Women with a urethral catheter may find a lateral position more comfortable for intercourse. Since sexual activity is a difficult topic for many people to discuss, it will usually be up to the nurse to introduce it and encourage the discussion of problems.

CATHETER CHANGES

The interval between catheter changes should be geared to the individual patient's needs. Some people experience repeatedly blocked catheters and are best with a routine fortnightly change to pre-empt problems. Others may be safely left for up to six months with no problems. Usually, the first catheter will be changed after a fortnight, the next after one month, the interval being increased until that individual patient's limit of tolerance is found. Some nurses leave all catheters until problems develop. This may be fine in hospital, but in the community it is preferable to anticipate problems, as they will so often occur at night or over the weekend. It is a good idea always to leave a full catheter-change kit in the home so that, if a professional unfamiliar with the patient is called in, the correct replacement catheter is to hand and the patient does not have to receive hospital treatment.

Catheter removal

To remove a Foley catheter, the water is drawn out of the balloon with a syringe. The widespread practice of intermittent catheter clamping and release prior to catheter withdrawal, often called 'bladder training' and said to restore 'bladder tone', has no proven value. The bladder in most cases soon resumes normal filling and emptying, once the catheter is out, provided that fluid intake is adequate and the patient is allowed enough time, privacy and comfort in which to void. He should be warned that micturition may be uncomfortable at first and reassured that this is temporary.

If voiding has not been achieved within six hours of catheter removal, or if the bladder becomes distended or painful, an in-out catheter will remove the residual urine and allow a further chance for normal function to return. When a catheter has been removed in the home, the nurse must always check later that day, and again the next day, to see that the patient has resumed normal voiding.

The non-deflating balloon

Occasionally a catheter balloon will not deflate with a syringe. It is very important when inflating a balloon to use only sterile water and to be sure that no contaminants come into contact with the water (e.g. powder from sterile gloves). The inflation lumen is extremely narrow and easily blocked. If saline or other solutions are used, the solutes may precipitate out to block the lumen.

If the balloon will not deflate, it is *not* a good idea to attempt to burst it with extra water (it takes up to 100ml to burst a 5ml balloon, and up to 200ml to burst a 30ml one), as the trauma can damage the bladder mucosa and there is a high risk of leaving small particles of balloon behind. These particles will almost always form the nucleus for stone formation. Nor should the balloon be dissolved, for example with ether. Chemicals can cause an acute chemical cystitis and there is again a risk of some particles of balloon remaining inside the bladder.

The fault may be in the valve, so the inflation arm should be cut right across. If the water does not come out immediately, it should be left for up to twenty-four hours to deflate slowly. If the balloon still will not deflate, the inflation channel must be blocked higher up. Unless the nurse is very experienced with this problem, this is the time for urological referral. The urologist might burst the balloon using a long stilette via the inflation lumen. Alternatively, the balloon can be punctured under local anaesthetic via the perineum in men, or the vagina in women, or with X-ray control via the abdominal route. With all these methods the catheter and balloon must be examined very carefully, and if there is any suspicion that they are incomplete, the particles must be removed at cystoscopy.

All cases of faulty catheters should be reported for investigation to the manufacturer and to the DHSS, Scientific and Technical Division (see Appendix 2 for address).

CATHETER TEAMS

In the USA specialist catheter teams have been introduced into some hospitals with large numbers of catheterised patients, notably neurological units. In the UK the specialist catheter nurse has more often been community-based, usually liaising with a hospital urological unit (Ferrie et al., 1979). Such nurses have often greatly improved patient management by introducing planned regimes of catheter care, anticipating problems, and sorting out any problems in the patient's own home. Many patients, especially males, still have to make a trip to the hospital outpatient department for catheter changes, or to Casualty if the clinic is closed. Catheter teams can greatly reduce the need for repeated hospital visits, as well as providing continuity of care between hospital and community for the patient being discharged home with a catheter for the first time. Research is needed to evaluate further the cost-effectiveness and potential improvements in patient care from such specialist nurses.

CONCLUSIONS

The decision to catheterise must never be taken lightly and should always be made with both the benefits and risks in mind. One of the most important factors in the successful use of a catheter is good communication between all persons involved – patient, nurse and doctor. Written records should always be kept of catheter size, type, changes, and problems. As with any other aspect of nursing care, planned management rather than ad hoc intervention will benefit the patient.

The more the patient is involved in the care of his catheter the better. If he handles it confidently and without fear, his independence will be greatly enhanced (Blannin, 1982).

The catheter must always be there for a reason. Too often professional attention is focused on sorting out catheter problems rather than questioning, 'Why is it necessary?' If it causes more problems than it solves, take it out! There is still much to be learned about ideal catheter management. Much more research is needed before optimum management is available to all.

SUPRAPUBIC CATHETERS

A suprapubic catheter is a catheter inserted directly into the bladder via the anterior abdominal wall. It is always inserted by a medical practitioner in the first instance, either under general or local anaesthetic.

INDICATIONS

The suprapubic catheter is especially useful after pelvic or urological surgery where the patient might have difficulty in resuming voiding. The catheter can be clamped for a trial of voiding. If unsuccessful, the catheter can merely be unclamped again (so avoiding repeated urethral catheterisations (Hilton and Stanton, 1980). The suprapubic catheter is likewise useful in acute retention as voiding can be attempted without catheter removal.

The suprapubic catheter can be used for long-term drainage, especially in sexually active patients and those experiencing problems with urethral catheters. In some women the urethra may be closed surgically (Feneley, 1983).

THE CATHETERS

There are several makes of suprapubic catheter. Sizes range from 6 f.g. to 16 f.g. Some are secured to the abdominal wall by a stitch or medical adhesive; others have a balloon for retaining the catheter (Figure 15.8). Foley catheters may also be inserted suprapubically.

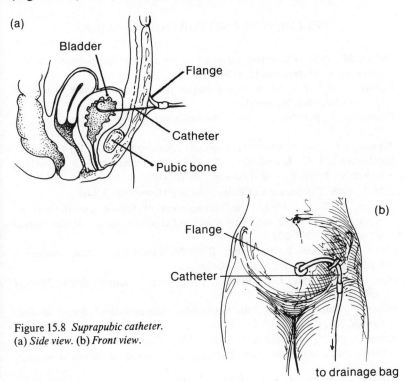

Figure 15.8 *Suprapubic catheter.*
(a) *Side view.* (b) *Front view.*

MANAGEMENT

Suprapubic catheters are associated with lower infection rates than urethral catheters. This may be because the urethral defence mechanisms are left intact and the entry site is relatively easy to keep clean. The entry site should be inspected daily and gently cleaned with mild antiseptic (e.g. 0.5% aqueous chlorhexidine), and kept covered with a sterile dressing. Otherwise management is the same as for urethral catheters: the same bags may be used and the same instructions given to patients. If the catheter becomes heavily infected, it will often block easily if a small size has been used. If the skin round the puncture site becomes infected, systemic antibiotics may be necessary.

293

Once the channel is established, the catheter can usually be easily changed by medical or nursing staff via the original channel, without further anaesthetic. When the suprapubic catheter is no longer needed it can simply be removed. The opening in the abdominal and bladder wall normally closes spontaneously without complication.

REFERENCES AND FURTHER READING

Bielski, M., 1980. 'Preventing infection in the catheterised patient'. *Nursing Clinics of North America*, 15, 4, 703–713.

Blandy, J. P., 1981. 'How to catheterise the bladder'. *British Journal of Hospital Medicine*, 26, 58–60.

Blannin, J. P., Hobden, J., 1980. 'The catheter of choice'. *Nursing Times*, 76, 48, 2092–2093.

Blannin, J. P., 1982. 'Catheter management'. *Nursing Times*, 78, 11, 438–440.

Brocklehurst, J. C., Brocklehurst, S., 1978. 'The management of indwelling catheters'. *British Journal of Urology*, 50, 102–105.

Cule, J., 1980. 'Forerunners of Foley'. *Nursing Mirror*, 150, 5, i–vi.

Feneley, R. C. L., 1983. 'The management of female incontinence by suprapubic catheterisation, with or without urethral closure'. *British Journal of Urology*, 55, 203–207.

Ferrie, B. G., Glen, E. S., Hunter, B., 1979. 'Long-term catheter drainage'. *British Medical Journal*, 2, 1046–1047.

Flynn, J. T., Blandy, J. P., 1980. 'Urethral catheterisation'. *British Medical Journal*, 281, 928–930.

Hilton, P., Stanton, S. L., 1980. 'Suprapubic catheterisation'. *British Medical Journal*, 281, 1261–1263.

Kennedy, A. P., Brocklehurst, J. C., 1982. 'The nursing management of patients with long-term indwelling catheters'. *Journal of Advanced Nursing*, 7, 411–417.

Kennedy, A. P., Brocklehurst, J. C., Lye, M. D. W., 1983. 'Factors related to the problems of long-term catheterisation'. *Journal of Advanced Nursing*, 8, 207–212.

Leonard, P., 1980. 'Catheters – a basic guide'. *Nursing Times, Community Outlook*, 76, 15, 104–105.

Platt, R., Polk, B. F., Murdock, B., Rosner, B., 1982. 'Mortality associated with nosocomial urinary tract infection'. *New England Journal of Medicine*, 307, 11, 637–642.

Smart, M., Ali, N., 1980. 'Long-term indwelling catheters – questions nurses ask'. *Nursing Times, Community Outlook*, 76, 15, 107–115.

Warren, J. W., Muncie, H. L., Jr., Bergquist, E. J., Hoopes, J. M., 1981. 'Sequelae and management of urinary infection in the patient requiring chronic catheterisation'. *Journal of Urology*, 125, 1–8.

Chapter 16

The Nurse and the Continence Adviser

CONTINENCE – EVERY NURSE'S BUSINESS

Almost every nurse, midwife and health visitor regularly encounters incontinent people in her everyday practice. Incontinence may not be the reason for the initial professional contact, but it is the nurse's duty to elicit any health-care problems from her patient or client and to plan nursing care to help resolve these problems.

What better opportunity to promote continence than a health visitor's child development check visit, when she can emphasise to the mother the value of preventive pelvic-floor exercises, not just immediately post-natally but on a continuous basis? And who better to pick up the early signs of problems, in the privacy of the patient's own home? And what an ideal time to teach the principles of good bladder and bowel care, thereby possibly preventing problems for the next generation. Who is more likely to be the first to detect an old lady's incontinence than the district nurse who visits weekly to dress her leg ulcers? Each visit need not take much longer if the nurse spends a few minutes giving advice on bladder training. There is no better time to start bladder rehabilitation than during hospital admission for an acute disease or injury that may cause incontinence. Yet the fact remains that many opportunities to prevent, detect, treat or manage incontinence are missed by nurses because of lack of knowledge, awareness or motivation. Many nurses still feel that incontinence is someone else's responsibility, or that it is inevitable and irreversible.

The nurse must give every patient the opportunity to discuss continence problems. She herself must not be embarrassed, and should be able to talk about excretion frankly and openly. The patient will soon detect any reticence on the part of the nurse and may then lack courage to broach the subject. To encourage discussion, the nurse must feel confident in her own knowledge and ability to tackle the problem; those who are unsure can easily discourage any such discussion. If the patient says, 'I expect it's my age', and the nurse simply agrees, the subject will end there rather than being fully explored in an attempt to find a remedy. The nurse who simply accepts incontinence, or feels helpless to do anything about it, will transmit those feelings to her patient.

As co-ordinator for services to the incontinent, the nurse must be fully aware of which services are available locally and how to arrange them, and if services do not exist, how and whom to pressurise for their provision. Other members of the multidisciplinary team often need stimulating into action by suggestions or prompts. The nurse must also be sure that her actions neither overlap nor leave gaps in patient care.

Most education on incontinence is delivered piecemeal during nurse training as part of basic nursing care (skin care and pressure-sore prevention), or as part of the teaching of a medically-orientated speciality, such as urology or gynaecology. Seldom is incontinence singled out and treated as a separate nursing subject. Teaching on the topic has improved since geriatric nursing has become compulsory for student as well as pupil nurses, but there are still some schools of nursing where it is given scant attention. It is often presumed that nursing care for incontinence is something that learners can pick up as they go along, and will be able to integrate for themselves into a co-ordinated care plan. Presumptions are made that learners will acquire information on aids during community experience (which, however, is often only a few days and may be in a District with very poor provisions), and on catheters during urology (where there may be no long-term catheters anyway). Some textbooks offer sound information and advice (especially in geriatric nursing). However, many of the older standard texts offer very limited information and reinforce the opinion that incontinence care can do little more than prevent skin breakdown.

Education should not stop at the end of training. It needs to be an ongoing activity, especially in a subject where there are so many new developments in nursing techniques. Many post-basic courses now include continence and incontinence as a topic. Updating by study days, seminars and exhibitions is growing in popularity. Several good visual aids are available (see under References) – especially useful where local expertise is limited. For the nurse who wishes to explore the subject in more depth the English National Board Course 984, 'The Promotion of Continence and Management of Incontinence', offers the opportunity to gain detailed knowledge.

The trend of modern nursing is towards individualised total patient care. It is most important that bladder and bowel management should be fully integrated with the rest of the care that a patient receives, and that continence is not fragmented off and treated separately. Few, if any, of the suggestions for nursing interventions made in this book are beyond the capability of any nurse who has the appropriate knowledge and training. Bladder training, pelvic-floor exercises, selection of an aid, intermittent catheterisation, modification of the environment, bowel management – all of these are well within her or his capability. Nor is there anything very difficult in making an assessment of the problem, given adequate time and an understanding of what information is needed.

If continence is every nurse's business and all should be able to deal with it, what role is there for the specialist 'continence adviser'? Is there a need for a specialist nurse? Not for the day-to-day management, perhaps, nor for the assessment and treatment of every incontinent person, but as a clinical support for nurses who have incontinent patients, as catalysts for improved care and co-ordination of services, and as educators and researchers.

THE DEVELOPMENT OF CONTINENCE ADVISERS

A look at how these specialist posts have arisen may provide an understanding of the way in which such nurses function today.

Nearly all specialist posts have started within the past decade. Most of the first posts were created in the context of research-based urodynamic clinics. Often a nurse was appointed, usually on a research grant, to assist with urodynamic investigations and to look after the patients during the tests. From fulfilling this limited role, many nurses became interested in the nursing aspects of incontinence and sought information on conservative methods of management and aids. Such information was hard to obtain because so little had been written. This prompted some nurses to conduct their own research and to write articles. A few obtained research grants in their own right to conduct nursing research on incontinence. Most were asked to give talks and lectures to various groups of professional and lay people.

As the concept of the clinical nurse specialist has gained increasing popularity within the nursing profession, so the idea of having a continence adviser has spread. At first it was usually one of these urodynamic/research nurses who had proved her value locally and who was then taken on to health authority staffing when the research grant ran out, so as not to lose that expertise. Increasingly, as word has spread about the value of these specialists, new posts have been created separately from any research or urodynamic links.

In 1983, there were forty full-time nurse specialists employed in the UK (Incontinence Action Group, 1983). There were probably an equal number who have the role as part of wider responsibilities (e.g. as part of a nursing officer role in community or geriatrics, or added to responsibility for stoma care). Growth has been haphazard with no central co-ordination or guidance, and this is reflected in the great variety of different posts that now exist. Even the names vary: from 'incontinence adviser' or 'nurse specialist for the promotion of continence', to 'sister for research into incontinence'. Grading varies from staff nurse, through sister, to senior nurse. There is little agreement about what such a person should do – there is no standard job description and expectations vary enormously. Some advisers are employed by a hospital, some by the community nursing services. Some are jointly funded. Some cover one specific sphere (e.g. one hospital, handicapped children or the elderly). Others have responsibility for a whole Health District, or even Region. Some work as teachers or resource-persons only, others see patients full-time, most do both. Some of the part-time post-holders are in the almost impossible position of having responsibility for incontinence added to other pre-existing responsibilities, with no extra time or resources allocated.

Too many continence adviser posts have been set up without adequate planning or resources. It has almost become a bandwagon, with a District Health Authority thinking they need one, setting aside a salary and an office, and expecting the new adviser to get on with an ill-defined task. Many have been limited-time projects, thus creating tremendous pressure on the adviser to produce 'results', without any knowledge of what criteria will be used for assessing success, and what 'results' she was aiming to produce. Calling someone an 'adviser' does not create an expert, and very careful thought should be given to the job description, funding and medical back-up before an appointment of this kind is made.

A few advisers have become overwhelmed by case-load work and have little time left to advise and teach. The Incontinence Action Group Report (1983) has recommended that at least one continence nurse adviser be appointed in each Health District. Before this happens, much thought needs to be given to what they should be doing.

THE SCOPE OF A CONTINENCE ADVISER

Most advisers in post fulfil all or most of the role outlined below. A detailed interpretation of the job would need to be adapted to local circumstances, and not be defined so rigidly as to restrict the development of the individual post-holder's interests and activities. However, any job description should contain some of the following.

Assessment and management of patients
The adviser will see individual patients to assess and manage their incontinence, and referrals will usually be taken from other professionals. In some situations a self-referral clinic may also operate. Where the referral is from a nurse, the adviser should be used for advice only, and not be expected to take over the management. The ideal situation would be a joint assessment with the referring nurse, collaboration over the formulation of a care plan, advice and support during implementation and help in evaluating its impact. The adviser should not (indeed cannot) expect or encourage referral of every incontinent patient, because of the numbers involved. The referring nurse should be taught how to carry out a basic assessment and encouraged to try the obvious remedies first, only referring problematic cases for advice. The adviser should not encourage the patient's own nurse to hand over this aspect of care; the referring nurse must retain responsibility for the patient's care, using the adviser as an outside pair of eyes which may view the problem from a fresh angle, and as a nurse with additional specialised expertise who may know of treatments or aids which have not yet been tried for the particular patient.

Some patients are referred who do not already have a nurse involved in their care. Provided that they are not in need of nursing care, but only require incontinence advice, the adviser will usually accept such people on to her own case-load. It is important that the adviser should retain a small case-load, as it is difficult to advise when not currently practising clinically, and it is always desirable to have first-hand experience in using new methods before recommending and explaining them to other practitioners. This is probably most important in the sphere of aids, as so many look promising but the problems only become evident when they are in use.

As well as advising nurses on the management of individual patients, the adviser should be available to offer suggestions on general points of patient care, such as ward routines. Clinical nurses should be able to consult the adviser on the best in current concepts of patient management and promotion of continence. In fulfilling this role, the adviser has to tread very carefully. She will not be accepted if she arrives uninvited and criticises current nursing practice. It is best to start to implement changes gradually, introducing new ideas one at a time. There should not be an expectation of changing attitudes overnight, nor should unrealistic expectations be raised.

Involvement in urodynamic/incontinence clinics

Where a specialist clinic exists within a District, the adviser will benefit from close links with it. In some circumstances this will mean actually running the clinic in conjunction with medical and other staff. The adviser can participate in a joint medical and nursing assessment of the incontinent person, help with any urodynamic tests involved and explain the results, and participate in planning and carrying out treatments as appropriate. In some cases the adviser may be able to do a home assessment or liaise with other professionals involved to complete the assessment.

Even where another nurse is employed specifically to run the urodynamic clinic, the adviser will naturally maintain very close links with the clinic. Where there is no such clinic the adviser tends to have less support, and it can be very difficult to manage some patients without access to specialised investigations. Often the adviser will have a role in persuading someone (usually a urologist, gynaecologist or geriatrician) to set up such a service. This is not to say that an adviser cannot work without such a clinic, but that it is greatly preferable if there is one.

Teaching

Teaching should in general be the primary role of the adviser. It is obvious that each District would need dozens of advisers if all incontinent people were to be seen by a specialist. As most incontinence management is within the scope of a general nurse, with a little additional instruction, teaching other nurses is obviously the best use of the adviser's time. This should be achieved by teaching both learners and qualified nurses and in keeping trained staff updated by regular in-service training. Formal lectures, seminars, workshops, exhibitions and more informal meetings can all be used for education, as well as clinic visits and working with the adviser for a short period. Indeed, one of the best teaching opportunities is in the one-to-one situation of the joint assessment of a patient – the adviser can teach assessment skills which the referring nurse could then use in assessing her next incontinent person.

Teaching will not be confined to nurses. All professional groups can benefit from the adviser's knowledge and expertise. Medical students, qualified doctors (especially general practitioners and trainees in geriatric medicine), physiotherapists, occupational therapists, social workers and unqualified staff such as care assistants, nursing auxiliaries and home helps can all be helped greatly by an increased knowledge about incontinence. Teaching should obviously be geared to the background knowledge and respective needs of each group.

The patient and his relatives or carers will also benefit from teaching. This will usually be on an individual basis, but talks may also be given to groups (for example, Multiple Sclerosis Society, Association for Spina Bifida and Hydrocephalus, or pre-retirement courses and relatives' support groups). Advice on services, incontinence aids and management methods is often sought from the adviser by a diverse range of groups. Where the adviser wishes to, the teaching role can be extended to writing articles for the nursing and paramedical press in order to educate a wider audience.

Advisory service

The continence adviser should act as a resource and information centre. To this end she should keep up to date with all the current literature and trends in the field, and be available for consultation, whether by phone or in person, on all aspects of incontinence. This can range from recommending a new aid to giving a list of references on catheter management, from recommending a chart suitable for a particular use to advising on the latest research on urinary tract infections. Anyone planning a project on incontinence should be able to use books and papers for reference, and the adviser can help by building up a small reference library for general purposes. Samples of the range of aids should be kept so that people can see what is available, and where appropriate also to try them. Where space permits, a permanent exhibition of aids (especially those easily available in that District or for private purchase, if appropriate), with indications for use, is very valuable for staff training and updating.

When the adviser acquires new information she has the responsibility to disseminate it to all other professionals for whom it is relevant. In some places this is done via an 'incontinence interest group', with one representative from each area meeting regularly to take back information, or by a regular news sheet; or it may be done on an ad hoc basis as information becomes available, or via a link nurse in each clinical unit.

The adviser is also available to advise at District or Unit level on all matters relating to continence, for example on Procedure Committees or a Purchasing Advisory Group.

Liaison with Supplies
Good liaison with Supplies Officers and the aids distribution service is vital. When selecting aids as stock items or for contracts, the adviser can form a link between users and purchasers and may need to organise product appraisal or even formal clinical trials. Often this liaison is formalised in a Supplies working group which would include nurse managers, representatives from other disciplines, administration and supplies staff. This work aims to ensure co-ordination within and between areas (e.g. community and hospital), and to ensure that the users (patients and nurses) receive the best possible supplies in a relevant selection and quantity. Waste can be minimised by decreasing over-ordering or inappropriate orders. When new items are introduced, the adviser will often help with training all staff involved in how to use them. This is essential to the success or failure of new products. For instance, if the new item is better, lasts longer, but is more expensive, the full benefit will not be gained unless staff are trained to leave it in use for longer periods.

Often nurses feel they do not have a channel of communication with purchasers, and feel that they have no control over the aids they receive. The adviser can open these communication channels, and help to ensure that the patient is actually getting what he needs to help him to be continent or to disguise his incontinence.

Research
There is a desperate need for research on the nursing aspects of incontinence. In most areas there is a complete absence of a well-researched basis for practice. If continence advice is to become a recognised and respected area of specialised nursing practice, it must become more research-based than it is at present. This is true at every level, from small-scale descriptive studies to major research projects.

Links with manufacturers
With so many companies involved in making or marketing incontinence aids, and so much research and development currently being undertaken, the continence adviser must maintain good links with industry. This can be of great mutual benefit. The nurse can tell the manufacturer of any faults in products, and suggest improvements or new items. Industry can then obtain sensitive feedback on product

performance and ideas for future developments. Progressive companies are willing to invest heavily in educational programmes and the production of information booklets and teaching aids, taking the view that the greater the awareness among professionals about incontinence, the greater the potential market for the better-quality products.

Miscellaneous

There are so many potential areas of interest for the continence adviser that it is not possible to list them all. A few of the more common interests include: linen loan services; links with mental handicap teams, enuresis clinics and school nurses; involvement in health education, for instance via the family planning or well-women clinics; teaching in day centres and luncheon clubs. Local circumstances and priorities will dictate how far the adviser can become involved in these and other activities, with a view to promoting continence or improving provisions for the incontinent.

THE DANGERS OF SPECIALISATION

It has often been argued that we do not need and should not have nurse specialists for incontinence. If every nurse were properly educated the specialist would be superfluous, so it is said. To the advocates of the nurse specialist, this assumes there will be some future Utopia where every nurse has the training, both basic and ongoing, to keep updated on every aspect of her practice. This is unrealistic, certainly in the foreseeable future.

Even then the adviser would be left with a case-load of patients and a urodynamic clinic to run. Incontinence is a subject which has so many facets that it is difficult to imagine how the general nurse could keep up with every new development. Certainly, at present, there is such a degree of ignorance that we are very far from that Utopia. The various liaison functions outlined above merit someone to represent the interests of the patient and of nurses.

Antipathy to the continence adviser has often arisen because people have recognised the mistakes of some of the earlier nurse specialities, and fear fragmentation of patient care. A minority of practitioners in other specialities did make mistakes early on, tending to divide up the patient's care, rather than sharing their knowledge and teaching other nurses how to manage their own patients. It is not difficult to see how a general nurse may resent various specialists coming in to provide one particular aspect of care, usually leaving the more 'boring' routine work to the general nurse. It is good that nurses have made a stand

and resisted dividing up their patients into a series of specialist tasks, and have defended their role in total patient care. However, this view of the specialist as a fragmenter is based on a misconception. The nurse must learn to use the adviser as necessary, but not to think that by doing so she can give up responsibility for continence.

The adviser strengthens the validity of her role if she will freely share the techniques she uses with the express purpose of enabling the general nurse to do without her next time. When mutual suspicion gives way to mutual understanding and respect, the adviser can make a significant contribution to improving nursing practice. Incontinence is too big a problem to be left to the specialist.

SUPPORT FOR THE CONTINENCE ADVISER

The post of continence adviser can be a lonely one, especially when first appointed, and adequate managerial and peer group support can make a great difference. Management support will usually come from a line manager, who must be prepared to back the adviser in requests for resources and in establishing her clinical credibility and authority. Peer support is found by meeting others in similar posts locally and sharing information and expertise. The Association of Continence Advisors was founded in 1981 with the aim of opening up communication channels between interested professionals. Membership is multidisciplinary and not confined to continence advisers. The Association holds one national conference a year, and a network of Regional branches meet on a more frequent basis locally.

With time, an increasing number of continence advisers have published descriptions of their work and clinics. These can be very useful for any newcomer who does not know quite how to approach the setting up of an entirely new service in a District Health Authority (Blannin, 1980; Brink et al., 1983; Harris, 1984; Norton, 1984; Rooney, 1982; Shepherd et al., 1982; White, 1982). There has also been a start in evaluating an advisory service, and although initial studies have perhaps raised more questions than they have answered, such research is essential if continence advice is to become a recognised clinical nursing speciality. Both cost-effectiveness and clinical efficacy remain to be conclusively demonstrated (Badger et al., 1983; Ramsbottom, 1982, 1983).

The continence adviser and the general nurse, whether in hospital or community settings, have a huge task on their hands. It seems true at present to say that many nurses are not delivering the optimum possible care to their incontinent patients, and that they need both advice on how to improve that care and support in implementing it. Many incontinent people, possibly the majority, have the potential to regain continence if accurately diagnosed and correctly treated. Many of those with intractable problems could be helped to live a fuller and more independent life by the use of appropriate management techniques. The continence adviser must work with all nurses, other professionals, and the incontinent person and his relatives, to increase awareness, knowledge and facilities for tackling and alleviating this most distressing condition.

REFERENCES AND FURTHER READING

Badger, F. J., Drummond, M. F., Isaacs, B., 1983. 'Some issues in the clinical, social, and economic evaluation of new nursing services'. *Journal of Advanced Nursing*, 8, 487–494.

Blannin, J. P., 1980. 'Towards a better life'. *Nursing Mirror*, 150, 12, 31–33.

Brink, C., Wells, T., Diokno, A., 1983. 'A continence clinic for the aged'. *Journal of Gerontological Nursing*, 9, 12, 651–655.

Harris, J., 1984. 'A positive step'. *Nursing Mirror*, 158, 7, 16–17.

Incontinence Action Group, 1983. *Action on Incontinence.* Kings Fund Centre, London.

Norton, C. S., 1984. 'Challenging speciality'. *Nursing Mirror*, 159, 19, xiv–xvii.

Ramsbottom, F., 1982. 'Is advice really cheap?' *Journal of Community Nursing*, May, 9–16.

Ramsbottom, F., 1982. 'Advising the nurse'. *Nursing Times*, 78, 5, 24–28.

Rooney, V., 1982. 'A question of habit'. *Nursing Mirror*, 154, 19, Community Forum, ii–vi.

Shepherd, A. M., Blannin, J. P., Feneley, R. C. L., 1982. 'Changing attitudes in the management of urinary incontinence – the need for specialist nursing'. *British Medical Journal*, 284, 645–646.

White, H., 1982. 'Setting up an advisory service'. *Journal of Community Nursing*, Sept., 4–6.

VISUAL AIDS

Visual aids are available for teaching purposes from the following companies (addresses in Appendix 1): Coloplast; KabiVitrum; Smith and Nephew; Squibb Surgicare.

A teaching package for district nurses, which includes some visual aids, is available from the Royal College of Nursing, Birmingham Centre.

APPENDIX 1: MANUFACTURERS AND SUPPLIERS

ACS Medical Ltd., Kestrel House, Garth Road, Morden, Surrey SM4 4LP.

Ancilla (UK) Ltd., 97 Macadam Road, Earlstrees Industrial Estate, Corby, Northants. NN17 2JN.

Bard, C. R. International Ltd., Pennywell Industrial Estate, Sunderland SR4 9EW.

Brevet Hospital Products, 16 Bridge Street, Caversham, Reading, Berks. RG4 7AA.

Cape Engineering Co., Birmingham Road, Warwick CV34 4TX.

Clos-o-mat Ltd., 2 Brooklands Road, Sale, Manchester M33 3SS.

Coloplast Ltd., Bridge House, Orchard Lane, Huntingdon, Cambs. PE18 6QT.

Dow Corning Ltd., Reading Bridge House, Reading, Berks. RG1 8PW.

Downs Surgical PLC, Church Path, Mitcham, Surrey CR4 3UE.

Eschmann Bros. and Walsh Ltd., Peter Road, Lancing, West Sussex BN15 8TJ.

Franklin Medical Ltd., P.O.Box 138, Turnpike Road, Cressex Industrial Estate, High Wycombe, Bucks. HP12 3NB.

Freeman, William, & Co. Ltd., Suba-Seal Works, Staincross, Barnsley, South Yorkshire S75 6DH.

Ganmill Ltd., White Gable Works, North Petherton, Bridgewater, Somerset TA6 6PY.

Headingly Scientific Services, 45 Westcombe Avenue, Leeds LS8 2BS.

Henleys Medical Supply Co. Ltd., Alexandra Works, Clarendon Road, Hornsey, London N8 0DL.

KabiVitrum Ltd., KabiVitrum House, Riverside Way, Uxbridge, Middlesex UB8 2YF.

Kanga Hospital Products, P.O.Box 39, Bentinck Street, Bolton BL1 4EX.

LIC Ltd., 129 Groveley Road, Sunbury on Thames, Middlesex TW16 7JZ.

Loxley Medical, Bessingby Industrial Estate, Bridlington, North Humberside YO16 4SU.

Martin Creasey Rehabilitation, 89 Clumber Street, Hull HU5 3KH.

Mölnlycke Ltd., Hospital Division, Southfields Road, Dunstable, Beds. LU6 3EJ.

Nicholas Laboratories Ltd., 225 Bath Road, Slough, Berks. SL1 4AU.

Nottingham Medical Aids Ltd., 17 Ludlow Hill Road, Melton Road, West Bridgeford, Nottingham NG2 6HD.

Pearson Technical Services, Redlingfield Road, Occold, Eye, Suffolk IP23 7PG.

Peaudouce (UK) Ltd., Rye Road, Hoddesdon, Herts.

Rocket Ltd., Imperial Way, Watford, Herts. WD2 4XX.

Smith and Nephew Medical Ltd., Woodlands Road, Birmingham B8 3AG.

Squibb Surgicare Ltd., Squibb House, 141–149 Staines Road, Hounslow, Middlesex TW3 3JB.

Thackray, Chas. F., Ltd. (Raymed), Viaduct Road, Leeds LS4 2BR.

Vernon-Carus Ltd., Penwortham Mills, Preston, Lancs. PR1 9SN.

Warne Surgical Products Ltd., Walworth Road, Andover, Hants. SP10 5BG.

Appendices

APPENDIX 2: USEFUL ADDRESSES

Age Concern (England), 60 Pitcairn Road, Mitcham, Surrey CR4 3LL.

Association for Spina Bifida and Hydrocephalus (ASBAH), 22 Upper Woburn Place, London WC1H 0EP.

Association of Continence Advisors (ACA), c/o Disabled Living Foundation (see below).

Colostomy Welfare Group, 38/39 Eccleston Square, London SW1V 1PB.

Department of Health and Social Security, Scientific and Technical Division (Supply Division), 14 Russell Square, London WC1.

Disabled Living Foundation (DLF), 380–384 Harrow Road, London W9 2HU.

Family Fund, P.O.Box 50, York YO1 1UY.

International Continence Society (ICS), c/o Hon. Sec. Mr. E. Glen, FRCS, Consultant Urologist, Southern General Hospital, Glasgow G51.

Multiple Sclerosis Society, 286 Munster Road, Fulham, London SW6.

Royal Association for Disability and Rehabilitation (RADAR), 25 Mortimer Street, London W1N 8AB.

Spinal Injuries Association (SIA), Yeomans House, 76 St. James Lane, London N10.

Sexual and Personal Relationships of the Disabled (SPOD), 286 Camden Road, London N7 0BJ.

Urinary Conduit Association, 36 York Road, Denton, Manchester.

APPENDIX 3: GENERAL FURTHER READING

BOOKS FOR PROFESSIONALS

Association of Continence Advisers, 1984. *Directory of Aids*, (second edition). ACA, London. Comprehensive catalogue of the aids available on the UK market, with notes on selection.

Browne, B., 1978. *Management for Continence*. Age Concern, Mitcham, Surrey. Practical advice for those working in Residential Care for the elderly.

Caldwell, K. P. S., (ed.), 1975. *Urinary Incontinence*. Sector Publishing, London. Medical textbook covering anatomy and physiology, investigation, and treatment.

Disabled Living Foundation, 1981. *Incontinence Bibliography*. Reedbooks, Chertsey. Comprehensive bibliography of articles and books published from 1974–1980.

Mandelstam, D., (ed.), 1980. *Incontinence and its Management*. Croom Helm, Beckenham. Contributions by members of different disciplines on aspects of management.

Smith, P., Smith, L., (in press). *Continence – Normal and Delayed Development*. Croom Helm, Beckenham.

Stanton, S. L., 1977. *Female Urinary Incontinence*. Lloyd-Luke, London. Medical textbook covering causes, investigation and treatment.

Stanton, S. L., (ed.), 1978. *Clinics in Obstetrics and Gynaecology: Gynaecological Urology*. W. B. Saunders, London. Medical contributions on many aspects of female incontinence.

Stanton, S. L., (ed.), 1984. *Clinical Gynaecologic Urology*. C. V. Mosby Company, St. Louis. Comprehensive text on all aspects of female incontinence.

Willington, F. L., (ed.), 1976. *Incontinence in the Elderly*. Academic Press, London. Medical textbook.

BOOKS FOR THE GENERAL PUBLIC

Disabled Living Foundation. *Notes on Incontinence*. DLF, London. Practical advice for the patient or his carers.

Feneley, R. C. L., Blannin, J. P., 1984. *Incontinence: Patient Handbook*. Churchill Livingstone, Edinburgh and London. Clear description of causes, treatment, and self-help.

Mandelstam, D., 1977. *Incontinence: a Guide to the Understanding and Management of a Very Common Complaint*. Heinemann, London. Practical advice for the sufferer.

Meadow, R., 1980. *Help for Bedwetting: Patient Handbook*. Churchill Livingstone, Edinburgh and London. Advice for enuretics of all ages.

Montgomery, E., 1983. *Regaining Bladder Control*. Wright–PSG., Bristol. Exercises, especially for stress incontinence.

Morgan, R., 1981. *Childhood Incontinence*. Heinemann Medical Books, London. For parents or the older child with day or night wetting or soiling.

ARTICLES, REPORTS, REVIEWS

Age Concern & Disabled Living Foundation, 1979. *Improving Services for the Incontinent Adult*. Age Concern, Mitcham, Surrey. Survey and recommendations for services.

Disabled Living Foundation. *A Checklist and Guidelines for Professional Staff*. DLF, London.

Incontinence Action Group, 1983. *Action on Incontinence*. Kings Fund Project Paper, Kings Fund Centre, London. Review of current services and training of professionals, with recommendations for improvements.

International Continence Society. Proceedings of annual conferences published in the form of abstracts of scientific papers presented.

Norton, C. S., 1983. 'Training for urinary continence'. In: Wilson-Barnett, J., (ed.), *Patient Teaching. Recent Advances in Nursing* series. Churchill Livingstone, Edinburgh and London. Review of nursing literature and research on teaching patients to be continent.

Norton, C. S., 1985. 'Eliminating'. In: Redfern, S., (ed.), *Nursing Elderly People*. Churchill Livingstone, Edinburgh and London. Review of nursing literature and research on planning care for urinary and faecal elimination in elderly patients.

Nursing, 1980 (Oct.). 'Urinary Elimination'. Issue devoted to urinary elimination.

Nursing Times, 1984. Supplement: 'Continence', 80, 14.

Royal College of Nursing, 1983. *The Problem of Promoting Continence*. RCN, London. An account of 16 regional study days convened to discuss services and needs.

Willington, F. L., 1976. *Incontinence*. Nursing Times publication, London. Collection of articles published in *Nursing Times*.

Index

acute care 201-2, 268
admission 204
ageing (effect on
    continence) 144-50
aids for incontinence 35, 71,
    72, 74, 83, 139, 153, 217,
    219-46: assessment
    224-6; continence adviser
    299, 301, 302-3; delivery
    198; disposal 200-1;
    faecal 263; laundry 200;
    selection 219-24; supply
    194, 222-4
alarms: enuresis 100-5, 217;
    forgetful 196; pants 97, 105,
    216; toilet bowl 215,
    216-17; vibrating 103
anger 156
antibiotics 77, 145:
    catheter 280, 282, 283,
    287; intermittent
    catheterisation 188;
    neurogenic bladder 178
anticholinergic drugs 76,
    100, 286
anxiety 25, 37, 54, 82
artificial sphincter 79, 138
assessment (nursing)
    27-45: aids 224-6;
    behavioural 155-8; by
    continence adviser
    299-300; elderly 152;
    faecal incontinence 257,
    258-9, 266; home 192-3;
    neurogenic 177; residential
    care 205
Association of Continence
    Advisors 304
atonic bladder: causes 13,
    17, 176; drug therapy 77;
    elderly 148-9; post-
    micturition dribble 135;
    symptoms 34, 54;
    urodynamics 48, 55, 62-3
atrophic urethritis/vaginitis
    20, 33, 34, 39, 54, 71, 77,
    146-7, 286
attention-seeking 25, 151,
    156, 213-14
attitudes 6-7, 28, 37, 142-4,
    155, 203-4, 209, 216, 262,
    264, 300

bathing 70, 194, 197, 275,
    282, 284
bedpads 157, 222, 244
bedpan 169, 170, 255
beds 39, 150, 195, 202:
    protection 243-6
bedwetting - see nocturnal
    enuresis

behavioural assessment 37,
    80: charting 42-3; EMI
    43, 155-8; faecal
    incontinence 266; mental
    handicap 213-15
behaviour modification 159,
    210-17, 265-6
bereavement 25, 151
bidet 166
biofeedback 92
bladder: age changes 145;
    baby 9-11; congenital
    abnormalities 106-7;
    dysfunction 14-17;
    investigation 46-65;
    normal 12-13;
    trabeculation 129, 145;
    transection 78; washouts
    282, 287-9
bladder neck: incision 189;
    obstruction 133; stenosis
    145
bladder instability - see
    detrusor instability
bladder training 40, 77,
    80-92: catheter 290;
    children 96-8, 99; at home
    196; institutions 206-7;
    neurogenic 178; post-
    prostatectomy 135
bottle 36, 167-9
bottom wiper 166
bowels 18-19, 35, 74, 133,
    249-50, 255-6

carcinoma: bladder 20, 34,
    287; bowel 250, 253, 255,
    262; prostate 132, 147
carers 13, 25, 38, 54, 68-9,
    141-2, 154: aids 219; EMI
    156, 159; at home 192,
    194-7; intermittent
    catheter 182
catheter 267-94: acute care
    202; -cramps 286; elderly
    145; fluids 74; Foley
    267-92; -introducer 276;
    neurogenic 180, 189, 190;
    skin care 71; suprapubic
    292-4; -teams 291;
    terminal care 153;
    urethral stricture 132;
    urine specimen 282-3;
    urodynamics 50, 55
cerebrovascular accident 14,
    174-5, 251-2
charts 35, 40-5: bladder
    training 82-90, 91, 97; EMI
    157, 206; enuresis alarms
    103-4; neurogenic 178;
    star chart 100-1

checklist: defaecation
    257-9; urinary
    incontinence 29-45
childbirth 35: faecal
    incontinence 250-1, 262;
    fistula 121; pregnancy
    122-3; exercises 114;
    stress incontinence 113
children 93-108: disabled
    182; faecal incontinence
    263-5; intermittent
    cathetherisation 182;
    mentally handicapped
    208-18
clothing 24, 79: catheter
    277-8; disabled 171-3;
    elderly 150; laundry
    198-200; manual dexterity
    36; mental handicap 214;
    odour 72; post-micturition
    dribble 133; replacement
    198
colostomy 263
commode 143, 166-7, 195
community: -care 192-201,
    209; -Mental Handicap
    Team 209, 215;
    -Psychiatric Nurse 80, 155
confused patient 24, 37, 43,
    54, 129, 148, 154-60: aids
    229-30; catheter 272-3,
    287; faecal incontinence
    253, 255, 265-6; fluids 73,
    149
congenital abnormalities
    106-7, 113, 250, 264
constipation 18-19, 35, 39,
    73, 253-62: catheter 284,
    285; child 100, 264; elderly
    144, 149; long-stay 205
continence: faecal 247-9;
    toilet training 94-6;
    urinary 10-13
continence adviser 295-305
Crede 179-80
cystocele 115
cystodistension 78
cystometry 50-65:
    biofeedback 92;
    neurogenic 177;
    prostate 130
cystoscopy 130, 132, 133

defaecation 247-66
dehydration 33, 39, 73, 149,
    194, 253, 254
delivery (pads) 198
dementia 24, 37, 54, 91, 148,
    154-60, 174-5, 204, 206,
    225, 238, 251-2, 255,
    265-6

denial 37, 157, 193, 225
deodorants 73, 197
depression 25, 37: elderly 149; EMI 154; faecal incontinence 253, 255; long-stay 204-5
detrusor hypertrophy 17, 129, 145
detrusor instability 13, 14-15, 17, 20-1, 25, 33, 34, 54, 109, 121, 122, 135, 139, 145, 148, 153: bladder training 81-90; catheter 272, 286-7, 288; drug therapy 75-7; neurogenic 174-5, 177-8, 191; prostate 129-30; surgery 78; urodynamics 55, 56-7, 60-1
detrusor-sphincter dyssynergia 16, 148, 176, 177, 191
diabetes 17, 20, 39, 42, 54, 148-9, 154, 175, 177, 253, 255
diaper-style pads 154, 217, 234-5, 246
diarrhoea 250: spurious 253, 264
diazepam 19, 189
diet 70, 80, 114, 194, 249, 253-4, 257, 262
disabled 21, 36, 54, 75, 162-73, 204: carers 194-7; financial allowances 195; mental handicap 208; neurogenic 174
discharge from hospital 193-4
disposal of aids 164, 200-1, 225, 235
distance to lavatory 151
district nurse 193, 195, 197, 222, 225, 297
diuretic 19, 20, 33, 78, 149, 205
doctor, role of, 27, 75-9, 197, 202, 275
drainage bag: appliances 241-3; catheter 276-9, 281-2, 283, 284-5; penile sheath 239
draw-sheets 244, 245
dribble pouch 135, 236-7
dribbling incontinence 13, 54, 96, 107, 129
drip-type urinal 241
drug therapy: as cause 13, 19-20, 22-3, 35, 149; as treatment 75-8, 81, 100,

133, 135, 147, 152, 153; constipation 253, 255, 257; diarrhoea 250; neurogenic 177-8, 189; laxatives 260-1
dysuria 34, 98

ectopia 107
ectopic ureter 107
elderly 14, 18, 81, 141-61, 253, 255-6
elderly mentally infirm 154-60, 204
electromyelogram (EMG) 177
emotions 13, 24-5, 151-2
encopresis 264
encrustation (catheter) 273-4, 288-9
endocrine disorders 13, 20
enemas 252, 257, 260-1
English National Board Course 296
enuresis – see nocturnal enuresis
environment 13, 24, 38-9, 54, 72-3, 75: disabled 162-3; elderly 150-1; EMI 154-5, 158; faecal incontinence 253, 254, 262; home 197; long-stay 202-3, 204, 206
epispadias 106
eyesight 24, 36

faecal impaction 13, 18-19, 35, 39, 54, 130, 252-62: catheter 289; child 264; EMI 154, 266
faecal incontinence 35, 153, 205, 247-66: aids 234, 244, 245
faradism 79, 119
feet 24, 36
financial benefits/costs 3, 80, 165, 195, 198, 199-200, 208-9, 224, 226
fistula 121-2, 154
flow rate 46-9, 130
fluid intake 21, 33, 35, 42, 70, 72, 73-4, 83, 206: catheter 284, 288, 290; constipation 254, 262; elderly 149-50; enuresis alarm 105; as reward 214-5
frequency 12, 13, 14, 16, 17, 18, 32-3, 42, 54, 73, 81-90, 96-7, 123, 129, 135, 178, 206

general practitioner 197, 222
genuine stress incontinence 13, 16, 33, 54, 109-21, 145, 180: bladder training 81; child 98; drug therapy 77; male 135-8; surgery 78, 119-21; urodynamics 49, 55, 58-9
Geriatric Visitor 198
giggle incontinence 98, 113
grab rails 165

habit retraining 43-4, 91
haematuria 34, 129: catheter 270, 272, 285, 287, 288; intermittent catheter 186, 187, 188
haemorrhoids 129, 253, 255
handwashing 143, 188, 281-2
health visitor 94, 100, 114, 123, 193, 198, 265, 295
hesitancy 34, 129
home care 192-201: catheter 283-5, 290; mental handicap 208, 217
home help 72, 194, 195, 198, 199, 225
hospital 201-7: acute 201-2; discharge 193-4; long-stay 202-7; mental handicap 209
hygiene 36-7, 72, 194, 225, 230, 243
hypospadias 106-7
hypothyroidism 253, 255
hysterectomy 119, 120

imipramine 76, 77, 100
immobility 13, 21, 36, 54, 79, 149, 154, 162, 178, 205, 225, 250, 253, 254, 255, 256, 257, 262, 288
implantable devices 136-8
individualised care 158, 201, 205, 206-7
individualised training 212-13
infection – see urinary tract infection
interferential therapy 79, 119
intermittent catheterisation 152-3, 180-9, 190, 191, 283
investigation: faecal incontinence 256-7; neurogenic 177; urinary incontinence 27-65

Kaufman urinary prosthesis 136

laundry 39, 72, 80, 194, 198–200, 225, 235, 245

lavatories 24, 38–9: disabled 162–6; disposal 200–1; elderly 151; EMI 155, 157; faecal incontinence 254, 257; home 197; long-stay care 202–3

laxatives 77, 255–6, 257, 260–1, 262, 264

long-stay care 5–6, 13, 38, 91, 151, 154–60, 201, 202–7, 209, 212, 234, 245, 253

male appliances 236–43

manual dexterity 24, 36–7, 167, 170, 171: aids 225, 229, 233, 238

manual expression 34, 179–80

mattress cover 72, 243–4

menopause 113, 146

menstrual cycle 111

mental handicap 24, 37, 54, 105, 208–18, 265

mental impairment 13, 24, 37, 54, 80, 91, 148, 154–60, 225, 265–6

micturating cystogram 133

micturition 9–12

mobility – see immobility

motivation 24, 198

Multidisciplinary Team 2, 27, 79–80, 202, 210, 216, 296

multiple sclerosis 21, 54, 174, 175, 178, 189, 251–2

neo-urethra 79, 121

neurogenic bladder 14, 16, 17, 54, 174–91: bladder neck obstruction 133; elderly 148; mental handicap 208

neurogenic faecal incontinence 251–2, 257

nocturia 14, 32, 54, 74, 129

nocturnal enuresis 14, 34, 54, 75, 98–105: aids 233, 243–6; behaviour modification 159; fluids 74; mental handicap 216–17

nurse 1–2, 25: acute care 201–2; assessment 27–45, 224–6, 257, 258–9; attitudes 6–7; catheter 275, 291; and continence adviser 295–305; faecal incontinence 253, 255, 261, 262; home care 192–3,

197–8; intermittent catheterisation 152–3; long-stay care 202–7; management and advice 67–75; mental handicap 210, 216

occlusive devices: female 123–7; male 139–40

occupational therapist 79, 173, 198, 202

odour 37, 71–3, 194, 195, 197, 201, 220, 229, 243, 263

oestrogen: deficiency 20, 111, 146–7; therapy 77, 114, 145, 147, 286

outflow obstruction 13, 16–17, 18–19, 34, 54, 129, 133, 148: drug therapy 77; surgery 78; urodynamics 48, 55, 64–5

overflow incontinence 13, 16, 17, 18, 33, 34, 54, 81, 107, 109, 129, 133, 149, 176–7, 178, 182

overlearning 105

pads and pants 34, 35, 71, 122, 154, 160, 172–3, 198, 217, 219–35, 246, 263

paradoxical urination 157

paraurethral glands 270–1, 286

Parkinson's Disease 21, 149, 175, 255

passive incontinence 34, 54, 121

pelvic floor 110–119, 248–9, 262

pelvic floor exercises 79, 115–119: bladder training 84; children 98; faecal incontinence 251; post-natal 114; post-prostatectomy 135; pregnancy 123

penile clamp 139–40, 276

penile sheath 154, 189, 237–40, 281

penis and scrotum urinal 241, 243

perineometer 118

phenoxybenzamine 77, 133, 189

physical examination 39: at home 193; pelvic floor 115–17; prostate 129; rectal 253, 256, 262

physiotherapist 79, 114, 119, 173, 198, 202

post-micturition dribble 16, 34, 133–5

post-prostatectomy incontinence 54, 130, 135–8

precipitancy 33

pregnancy 120, 122–3

prescription 222, 237, 240, 243

pressure sores 70, 154, 165

prevalence of incontinence 4–6, 142

prevention: faecal incontinence 247; mental handicap 209; stress incontinence 114

prolapse: rectal 251; uterus/vagina 39, 54, 113, 115, 116, 119

propantheline 76, 286, 287

prostate: carcinoma 132, 147; catheter 281; elderly 144, 147–8; hypertrophy 16, 32, 54, 78, 128–31; post-micturition dribble 135; post-prostatectomy incontinence 135–8; prostatitis 133

psychiatrist 38, 69

psychological: assessment 37–8; elderly 151–2; faecal 264; support 68–9

psychologist 38, 69, 80, 155, 210

pubic pressure urinal 241–2

punishment 95, 212, 264

reality orientation 158–9, 203

rectocele 116

reflux of urine 55, 139, 180, 188

Registered Nurse for the Mentally Handicapped 210

regression 25, 155

renal function: catheter 280, 283, 289; children 96, 107; elderly 144; male 129–30, 131, 133; neurogenic 178, 189, 190

residential care – see long-stay care

residual urine 16, 17, 33, 51, 55, 129, 133: catheter balloon 272–3; elderly 144, 152–3; measurement 39, 77, 130; neurogenic 176, 178–90

retention 18, 34, 54, 77, 107, 109, 129, 176, 185, 190, 257, 268

retracted penis 139, 169, 225, 238, 241
rewards 96, 97, 100, 214–6, 264–5
ring pessary 124–5
rigid regimes 206
rocket foam pessary 124
Rosen prosthesis 137
routines (institutional) 155, 204, 205–7, 299

sacral neurectomy 78
sacral reflex arc 9–11, 14–15, 174–5, 176, 248
sedatives 19, 78, 149
self-catheterisation – see intermittent catheterisation
sensation (bladder) 12, 14, 17, 91, 148
septicaemia 283
services 4–5, 197–201, 225, 296
set interval toileting 91, 205–6
sexual function/ relationships 38, 69, 122: catheter 285, 289; congenital abnormalities 107; pelvic floor exercises 118; penile clamp 140; post-operatively 120; post-prostatectomy 131; ring pessary 125
skin care/problems 39, 70–1, 130, 147, 194, 195: aids 219, 225, 227; penile sheath 238–40; bed sheets 245
sling operations 119–21
smearing (faecal) 156, 264
smell – see odour
social network 38
Social Services 38, 197–200, 202
social worker 79, 198
spina bifida 173, 176, 182, 189, 265
spinal injury 54, 175, 176, 178, 180, 182, 189, 190–1, 251–2, 280
staff in long-stay care 203–4, 206–7, 212, 216
star chart 100–1
stoma care nurse 79, 190
stone (bladder) 20, 288, 291
stress incontinence (diagnosis) – see genuine stress incontinence

stress incontinence (symptom) 18, 33, 39, 54, 109–121, 123, 146: children 98; detrusor instability 55, 60–1; elderly 145; faecal 249, 250
supply of aids 217, 222–4, 225, 244, 302
suprapubic catheters 281, 283, 289, 292–4
suprapubic surgery 119–21
surgery 78–9: bladder neck obstruction 133; catheter 292; congenital abnormalities 106–7; elderly 152; faecal incontinence 251; neurogenic 189–90; pelvic floor exercises 116; post-prostatectomy incontinence 135–8; prostate 130–1; stress incontinence 119–21; urethral stricture 133

tabes dorsalis 175, 176
tampons 123–4
teaching: use of aids 226; catheter care 283–5; by continence adviser 299, 300–1; elderly 152; for hospital discharge 194; intermittent catheterisation 182–8; mentally handicapped 209; nurses 296; patient 68; pelvic floor exercises 115–8; spinal injury patients 191
terminal illness 153–4, 268
thyroid gland 20
toilet: frame 165; paper 165; tongs 166
toilet training 94–6, 208–17, 264
toileting programmes 80–91, 205–7
transfer (onto lavatory) 163–5, 195
tuberculosis 18

unstable bladder – see detrusor instability
upper motor neurone lesion 14, 54, 174–5
urethra: catheterisation 270–1; congenital abnormalities 106–7; dilatation 133; diverticulum 34; mucosal

prolapse 145; oestrogen 146–7; stricture 16, 78, 132–3, 270–1, 289; urethritis 132; valves 109
urethral pressure profile 55
urethral sphincter incompetence – see genuine stress incontinence
urethrotomy 78, 133, 189
urgency/urge incontinence 13, 14, 16, 18, 21, 33, 36, 54, 73, 75, 78, 109, 129, 135, 195: bladder training 81–90; children 96–7; elderly 150–1; institutional 206; neurogenic 174–5
urinals 36, 195: hand-held 167–71; male (body worn) 240–3; and pants 230; terminal care 153
urinary diversion 79, 107, 121, 138, 189, 190, 191, 283
urinary tract infection 13, 18, 20, 33, 34, 72, 73, 77, 129: catheter 272, 273, 279–83, 287, 288, 293; children 98, 107; elderly 144–5, 154; intermittent catheterisation 180–3, 188–9; neurogenic 178, 190; urine specimen 39, 72, 98, 130, 193, 282–3
urodynamics 45–65, 92, 110, 121, 130, 131, 152, 177, 297, 300

vaginal repair 119–21
Valsalva 179–80
videocystourethrography 55, 177
voiding difficulties (see also atonic/outflow obstruction) 34, 39, 54, 77, 96, 128–33: catheter 288; elderly 144, 145, 148, 149, 152–3; neurogenic 176, 177, 178–90; post-operative 292
voiding techniques 179–80, 189
voluntary incontinence 195
Voluntary Services 196, 197–8, 200

walking aids 36, 150
wheelchair 36, 163–4, 165, 171, 195, 230
wing-folded pad 233, 263